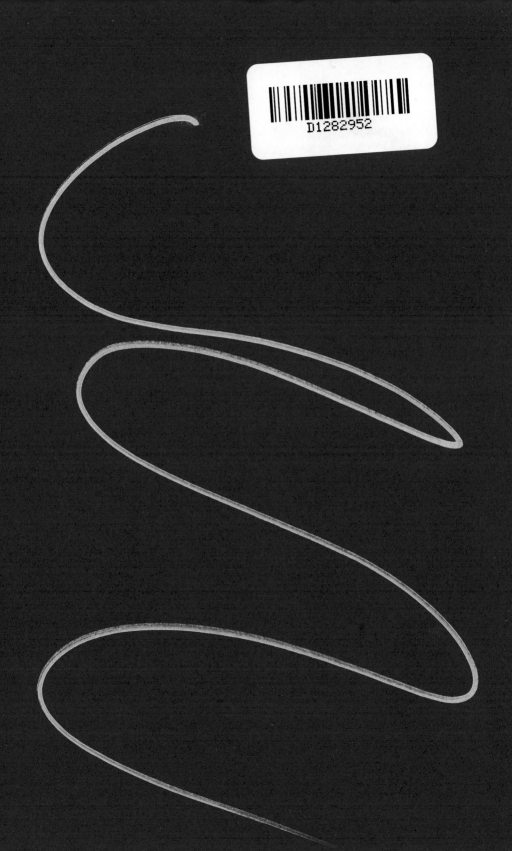

Committed

Committed

THE BATTLE OVER INVOLUNTARY PSYCHIATRIC CARE

DINAH MILLER, MD & ANNETTE HANSON, MD

FOREWORD BY PETE EARLEY

JOHNS HOPKINS UNIVERSITY PRESS

BALTIMORE

© 2016 Dinah Miller and Annette Hanson
All rights reserved. Published 2016
Printed in the United States of America on acid-free paper
9 8 7 6 5 4 3 2 1

Johns Hopkins University Press
2715 North Charles Street
Baltimore, Maryland 21218-4363
www.press.jhu.edu

Library of Congress Cataloging-in-Publication Data

Names: Miller, Dinah, author. | Hanson, Annette, author.
Title: Committed : the battle over involuntary psychiatric care / Dinah Miller, MD, Annette Hanson, MD.
Description: Baltimore : John Hopkins University Press, [2016] | Includes bibliographical references and index.
Identifiers: LCCN 2016002161| ISBN 9781421420783 (hardback : acid-free paper) | ISBN 1421420783 (hardback : acid-free paper) | ISBN 9781421420790 (electronic) | ISBN 1421420791 (electronic)
Subjects: LCSH: Mentally ill—Care—Moral and ethical aspects. | Mental health services—Moral and ethical aspects. | Involuntary treatment. | Psychiatric ethics. | BISAC: HEALTH & FITNESS / General. | MEDICAL / Psychiatry / General. | PSYCHOLOGY / Mental Illness.
Classification: LCC RC455.2.E8 M55 2016 | DDC 362.2—dc23
LC record available at https://lccn.loc.gov/2016002161

A catalog record for this book is available from the British Library.

Special discounts are available for bulk purchases of this book. For more information, please contact Special Sales at 410-516-6936 or specialsales@press.jhu.edu.

Johns Hopkins University Press uses environmentally friendly book materials, including recycled text paper that is composed of at least 30 percent post-consumer waste, whenever possible.

To the memory of my brother, Ross Miller.

—Dinah Miller

To my sister, for her undivided love and support, and to my brother, who showed me through his photography just how beautiful the world can be. And finally, to my parents, whose life lessons cannot be captured in words. I couldn't have asked for a better family.

—Annette Hanson

Contents

When should an individual be involuntarily committed?

For too many of us, this is not an abstract question. It is a painful and often horrific one for those who are committed against their will and for those who are responsible for involuntarily committing them.

In the pages that follow, Doctors Dinah Miller and Annette Hanson set out to examine involuntary commitment from every possible angle. This is a herculean task, not only because of the patchwork of differing statutes and procedures across the United States, but because of the strong opinions and emotions that always accompany forcing someone to accept psychiatric care.

This is not the first time these two Baltimore-based psychiatrists have collaborated, and it shows in the ease of their combined writing as they present research, profile patients, interview experts, and slip their personal observations seamlessly into this thought-provoking narrative. I first learned of the authors when I read *Shrink Rap: Three Psychiatrists Explain Their Work* (2011), which they penned with another colleague, Dr. Steven Roy Daviss. Soon I became an avid reader of the trio's blog, which bears the same title as their book and bills itself as "psychiatrists writing for psychiatrists," although it attracts a much broader audience.

Dr. Miller and I exchanged emails, and I came to admire her insatiable curiosity and her willingness to listen to other points of view. These traits are apparent throughout this book, especially in chapters 3 and 4. First, in chapter 3, we hear from mental health organizations and experts that are frequently quoted in news stories about involuntary commitment: the

National Alliance on Mental Illness, the American Psychiatric Association, and Dr. E. Fuller Torrey, who has spent decades calling for an easing of involuntary commitment laws and an increase in forced medication through assisted outpatient treatment. In chapter 4, we hear a different chorus. Miller startled members of the Church of Scientology by asking them to explain their antipsychiatry views and spent time listening to complaints from self-described mental health survivors who belong to MindFreedom, which opposes all forced psychiatric care. She interviewed Dr. Daniel Fisher, the psychiatrist and patient behind the National Empowerment Center, which advocates recovery with or without medication, and she talked with Ira Burnim at the Bazelon Center for Mental Health Law, whose founders questioned whether involuntary commitment could ever be justified. This willingness by Miller and Hanson to include the voices of critics hostile to their own profession gives readers a panoramic view that is vital in any serious discussion about the pros and cons of forced treatment.

Having introduced us to the major players in the debate, the authors zero in on what actually happens when someone is committed, explaining the hodgepodge of state laws and the use of restraints, electroconvulsive therapy, and medications. Because the US criminal justice system has come to play a major role in community mental health, there are chapters that focus on crisis intervention team training for the police (who may interact with more mentally ill Americans in a given day than psychiatrists do) and on mental health courts, guns, violence, and mass shootings.

That's a plateful for any book, but Miller and Hanson do a masterful job of illuminating each issue and giving it context. They don't skimp or oversimplify. There is more meat on the plate than salad.

While practical information gives *Committed* its spine, it is the emotions that we feel in reading patients' firsthand accounts that prick at the conscience and ultimately distinguish this book from some impersonal, analytical tome. That is one of the many reasons that this book should be read—because emotions lie at the heart of the involuntary commitment process, whether they are expressed in the angry voice of an unwilling patient or the anguished voice of a parent, spouse, sibling, friend, child, or professional caregiver.

These issues became real to me when I involuntarily committed one of my sons into a mental hospital. In my book, *Crazy: A Father's Search through America's Mental Health Madness*, he is identified by his middle name, Michael. He was an art student in Brooklyn when he began having a difficult time discerning reality from fantasy. A psychiatrist diagnosed him as having bipolar disorder with psychotic features and prescribed medication, but after several months Michael stopped taking his pills.

I was at work when I received a panicked call from my eldest son, who lived in Manhattan, telling me that Michael was "crazy." He'd been roaming the streets of New York City for five days with little sleep and hadn't bothered to eat because he believed God had ordered him to undertake a divine mission.

I rushed to Manhattan and persuaded Michael to return home with me to the northern Virginia suburb where I live. During that frantic ride, I pleaded with him to take his medication, but he screamed, "Pills are poison! Leave me alone!" His moods were herky-jerky. One moment, he would be laughing. Seconds later, he would break into gut-wrenching sobs.

"Dad, how would you feel if someone you loved killed himself?" he asked me.

I drove him to a hospital emergency room only to be told that there was nothing a doctor could do. At the time, state law in Virginia required a threat of "imminent danger" before a patient could be forcibly medicated, and the fact that my clearly psychotic son had not harmed either himself or me during our four-hour wait in an exam room showed there was no immediate threat. I was told to bring him back after he hurt himself or someone else.

Forty-eight hours later, Michael broke into a stranger's unoccupied house to take a bubble bath. The police arrested him and explained that my son would be taken to jail unless I told the examining psychiatrist that Michael had threatened me. If I said the magic words—"He threatened to kill me"—my son would get a one-way ticket to a psychiatric hospital, where an involuntary commitment hearing would be held the next morning.

This, then, was my choice. Lie and get him into treatment, or say nothing and watch him carted off to jail in handcuffs, completely confused and psychotic.

I chose to lie.

What happened next was a charade. A recent law school graduate appeared at the hospital 10 minutes before Michael's commitment hearing to interview half a dozen patients. I intercepted her. She was nice and polite. I wasn't. I insisted that she tell my son that he needed to voluntarily commit himself. Both the police and nurses had warned me that if Michael didn't voluntarily agree to treatment, he would be released and taken to jail. The administrative law judge who would determine my son's fate at this hearing was known for refusing to involuntarily commit anyone who didn't visually strike him as being dangerous—no matter how sick they were. In the hours that had passed since his arrest, Michael had calmed down.

My son's appointed attorney hastily interviewed Michael while I stood watch over her shoulder. His commitment hearing lasted less than four minutes. If you were to obtain access to his records, you would read that Michael voluntarily agreed to treatment.

But Michael and I both know better.

Now my son had to grapple not only with his mental illness, but also with feelings of betrayal and broken trust. At first, he refused to see me in the hospital. Later, he told me that he wanted "all of this" to go away. He wanted to turn back the clock to before he got sick. So did I.

After he was discharged, he didn't want to live with me. I eased my conscience by telling myself that I had not been given any choice. I had been forced to lie and to bully his attorney to keep him out of jail. Sometimes, I told myself, you have to risk having your child hate you in order to save him.

But it hurt. Badly.

Two years passed before my son again stopped taking his medication, and signs of his illness began to resurface. I called our county's mobile response crisis team and asked the dispatcher to send an evaluator to examine and counsel Michael.

"My son has stopped taking his medication," I explained.

"Is your son dangerous?" the dispatcher asked.

"No, not yet, but the last time this happened, he . . ."

"You can't judge him on what happened last time," the dispatcher snapped, interrupting me. "Call us when your son is dangerous."

A few days later, my ex-wife telephoned from her locked bedroom. She was afraid of Michael, who was living with her. I drove to her house and met Michael in the living room. He immediately ordered me to leave, and when I balked he threatened me and chased me into the street, returning to the house with his hands raised like a triumphant Rocky.

I called the dispatcher again and asked him to send a crisis unit.

"Is your son dangerous, or is he violent?" he asked.

"He is violent," I said.

"Oh, we don't come if someone is violent," he replied. "Call the police."

Three patrolmen arrived. When Michael ran from them, they shot him twice with a 50,000-volt Taser, hogtied him, and took him to a mental health center. I asked them to not file charges against him for refusing an order/resisting, and they agreed after I promised that I would get him involuntarily hospitalized.

Everyone's story is unique. But I share mine and Michael's to illustrate the complexity of what often happens when a person is psychotic and someone who loves them is trying to get them help. The decision to force someone into treatment is rarely as straightforward and clear-cut as it is presented by those who debate the issue in academic circles. Circumstances dictate actions. Choices often are not between right or wrong, but about which option will cause the least harm—as judged by an individual who knowingly risks damaging their relationship with the person who is sick but who does not have to endure the physical trauma of the decision.

This book does not sugarcoat what has to be one of the most difficult decisions in modern psychiatry, and we all benefit from that. In the final pages, you will find the authors' conclusions, and undoubtedly you will ask yourself, "What would I do?"

I've always found it interesting that how the involuntary commitment question is framed often elicits different reactions. Mention involuntary commitment, and many Americans immediately conjure up images of Nurse Ratched, of men in white coats armed with straitjackets, of lobotomies and zombie-causing medications, of being locked in a snake pit with no chance of freedom with your fate in the hands of sadistic doctors.

Because of our strong feelings about liberty, it is natural for Americans to declare that no one should be involuntarily committed as long as they are not hurting themselves or others. And as you read many of the accounts of those who were traumatized by being committed, you will likely agree.

Can you imagine what it must feel like to be taken from your friends and family, wrestled to the floor, stripped naked, confined in an empty room, and injected with powerful medications that knock you unconscious? Can you imagine the torture of being strapped to a hospital bed, unable to move for an hour, or four hours, a day? Can you imagine being treated as if you were some mindless child by strangers who claim to know what's best for you?

Who would want that?

But here's a different scenario for you to consider. Imagine your child, a loving and brilliant young art student in college. One morning, his friends deposit him on your doorstep and tell you that he is crazy. He is argumentative, refuses to eat or sleep, and is convinced that he needs to go immediately to the White House because God has given him a message for the president. Imagine watching him pace back and forth in front of a television with tin foil wrapped around his head to keep the Central Intelligence Agency from reading his thoughts. Imagine him being arrested because he has broken into a stranger's house to take a bubble bath. Imagine listening to someone you love scream at you, call you the enemy, tell you that he hates you. Imagine watching your son hit his own head to clear the voices inside his mind, which are screaming at him, telling him that he will die if he steps out of a car, taunting him to hurt himself, torturing him with thoughts of a girl he barely knew—but the voices say he impregnated. He must find the girl. *Hurry.* He has to go. *Where?* He doesn't know, but he must leave. *Immediately.* There's no time to explain. *Quick.*

Picture that, and remember that this is your son.

What would you do?

PETE EARLEY

Before We Get Started

On July 20, 2012, a gunman walked into a movie theater in Aurora, Colorado, and opened fire. Twelve people lost their lives that day, and 70 others were injured. For weeks after the tragedy, television, print, and social media were filled with images of the young shooter with his wide-eyed blank stare and tousled orange hair. Every videotaped court appearance and each tidbit of information about him was dissected as it emerged. Speculation abounded about the shooter's motivation, his psychiatric history, how much his college supervisors knew about his mental state, and what could have been done to prevent the tragedy.

Barely five months later, a different gunman killed his mother, then walked into the Sandy Hook Elementary School in Newtown, Connecticut, and shot 26 people dead before taking his own life. The Sandy Hook tragedy triggered another cycle of media speculation and public outrage. Aurora and Sandy Hook were added to the list of tragic place names: Columbine, Virginia Tech, Fort Hood, Isla Vista, the Washington Navy Yard, Tucson. Tragedies like these have captivated both the media and the public with a mix of horror and fear. To the general public it seems obvious that anyone who could do such a thing must be mentally ill, and the question gets asked repeatedly: Why don't we just commit people who are mentally ill so we don't have these tragedies?

President Barack Obama announced an initiative in 2013 to strengthen gun control laws as a way to prevent future violence. In addition to restricting access to weapons, there were proposals to loosen privacy protections for psychiatric patients, to enhance the sharing of information between mental health professionals and law enforcement, and to mandate the reporting of certain categories of psychiatric patients to the federal gun background-check database. To develop these recommendations, the president's commission gathered input from hunting enthusiasts, gun control lobbyists, crime victims, and law enforcement professionals. Oddly, people with mental disorders were not included in these discussions. Many states followed the proposals of the federal government and enacted their own legislation. For example, the New York Secure Ammunition and Firearms Enforcement (SAFE) Act was passed, mandating that mental health clinicians report any potentially dangerous psychiatric patient to the government.

The route to preventing mass murders was split into two paths—gun control or mental health reform—each hailed as a way to prevent yet another of these rare but terrifying events. When it came to talk about improving mental health care, the conversation invariably included options that would make it easier to mandate that people with problems get help. Groups in favor of looser civil commitment standards called for legislation that would make it less difficult to force people to get mental health care by making it easier to commit people to hospitals and easier for courts to order outpatient treatment. Proponents of *involuntary* care overlooked the facts that some perpetrators were already in treatment at the time of their crime and that some never gave any signals that they might be dangerous. They also did not acknowledge that some of the perpetrators had never been offered *voluntary* care.

Psychiatrists and psychologists, as well as their professional organizations, attempted to balance the public's concern with rationality and facts: the majority of people with psychiatric disorders never commit acts of violence; guns are more likely to be used to commit suicide than homicide; and people with psychiatric disorders are more often *victims* of crime than perpetrators. They also pointed out that substance abuse is a much greater risk factor for violence than is mental illness. Sadly, the facts did little to quell the public's fear of people with mental illness.

Proposals to expand involuntary psychiatric care inevitably lead to public discussions about the difficulty of predicting violent behavior, the limited funding for mental health services, the lack of access to voluntary care, and infringement on civil rights. Further, involuntary treatment is not always about preventing acts of violence; sometimes it's simply about getting treatment for someone who is very ill, whose disordered behavior might lead him or her to homelessness, jail, or death, and about the tragedy of wasted potential. Sometimes, it's simply about a family's heartbreak when a loved one becomes terribly ill.

Psychiatric illnesses are common. Interviews conducted with members of more than 18,000 households revealed that one out of every five people suffer from a psychiatric disorder in any six-month period, and nearly half of Americans suffer from an episode of mental illness at some point in their lifetime. Informed discussion about all these issues is difficult because there are so few people who are violent *solely* due to mental illness, and there are no statistics that can help to predict who is at risk of becoming violent. The federal government website www.data.gov lists all the publicly available data that the government routinely collects. There are more than 91,000 data sets with information about countless topics. There is information about average annual rainfall and daily temperatures, the number of annual motor vehicle accidents, and occupational injuries and fatalities. There are 9 data sets related to the price of pork and 13 related to the price of beans. There is even a data set devoted to the stomach contents of Alaskan fish. But there is no federal database that tracks the number of patients who are committed against their will to psychiatric units each year. This makes it difficult to examine the issues we write about in this book. Given the loss of liberty, the personal distress, and the stigma involved, this lack of data is astounding.

What we do know is that the number of state hospital beds has been reduced over the years. In 1955 there were 558,922 state hospital beds in the United States; by 2010 there were only 43,318 beds—a reduction of more than 90 percent during a period when the nation's population doubled. We also know that health insurers authorize admission only for the most dangerous of patients and for the shortest possible period of time, and that the typical length of a hospital stay—usually along the order of seven to ten days—is barely long enough to begin the process of stabilization for someone who is in a psychiatric crisis. We don't know how this concentration of the "sickest of the sick" affects the safety and therapeutic atmosphere of inpatient units, a patient's recovery, or a patient's willingness to seek hospitalization voluntarily in the future.

When it comes to discussions of forcing people to get psychiatric help, one thing is clear: the topic is touchy. Many people who have experience with mental illness—and many who don't—have strong opinions, and the topic quickly becomes a battleground populated by patients, families, mental health professionals, lawyers, advocates, and politicians. When we began collecting stories and data for this book, we quickly found that involuntary psychiatric care was a more sensitive topic than one might think. Some people were eager to take part, while others wanted nothing to do with the creation of this book. Simply put, not everyone was open to the concept of dialogue.

Many patients discuss their experiences with hospital commitment, sometimes in very public forums. Long after discharge, many remain very angry about being forced to get care and are haunted by their hospitalizations. They describe these experiences as degrading, frightening, and disrespectful. But some proponents of involuntary treatment dismiss patients' objections, deeming the treatment to have been necessary for the patients' own good when circumstances were dire and there seemed to be no other reasonable option.

What we also have heard is that there are people who won't get help because they are afraid they will be locked up, be stigmatized, lose their civil rights, or suffer other negative consequences. In a quick, unscientific online survey, we learned that 77 percent of our respondents who had previously been committed would not want to be committed again, even if they were imminently dangerous to themselves or others. Although our survey was not scientifically validated, we report the number because there simply are no other data.

We found this response to involuntary treatment perplexing. Shouldn't people who are ill, dangerous, or suffering from tormenting depression, delusions, or hallucinations be grateful that they were rescued from their misery and returned to a state of sanity? Shouldn't they be glad that no one was hurt or killed? Some are, but gratitude certainly doesn't seem to be the sentiment expressed by the majority of those who speak up. It is this divide that captured our attention and compelled us to write this book.

While psychiatrists practice at the center of this political and ethical maelstrom, the greatest impact of the changing social policy in the United States is obviously felt by patients, and we'll start with their voices. Some patients were grossly mistreated, while others were treated kindly but still felt anguish at their loss of freedom and control. As just one example of the stories that follow, a woman wrote to us about her experiences:

In 1998, I sought treatment at my Employee Assistance Program for depression. Over time it grew worse and I became suicidal. My therapist
asked if I would be willing to go into inpatient treatment and I agreed.
But she also started the involuntary commitment process so that when
I arrived at the hospital, I was handcuffed and placed in leg irons. All my
belongings were taken and I waited in a locked room for hours until the
sheriff came to transport me. I was led through the waiting area in handcuffs and chains and put in the back of a police car where I got to listen to
the deputies describe their hate for the "crazies" during the 45-minute ride
to a different hospital. Upon arrival there I was strip searched and placed
in isolation.

I was terrified throughout this whole process. I didn't understand why I
was being treated as a criminal when I agreed I needed help and I wanted
help. I am also a survivor of sexual assault and being strip searched was
horrible. I felt as though I had no value. I thought, wow, this is what everyone who has a psychiatric problem has to go through.

Would anyone be surprised if this woman hesitated to seek treatment the
next time she felt suicidal?

There are no studies that prove that involuntary treatment prevents
suicide, much less that such harsh treatment would be beneficial to anyone. Given the new push for loosening the restrictions on involuntary
commitment, stories like this are particularly difficult to hear.

The converging forces of fear-based legislation and financially driven
health care systems have taken American mental health care to a dangerous
point. People in need of inpatient psychiatric care experience unacceptable
delays even when they seek care voluntarily, and they face competition
for beds from patients who have been civilly committed. Psychiatric units
are increasingly filled with more potentially dangerous and unpredictable
patients.

When it comes to psychiatric treatment, and involuntary treatment in
particular, the battleground is busy. The discussions are animated and often
painful. On one side of the field, there are groups who oppose involuntary
psychiatric treatments under any condition; in fact, some groups oppose
psychiatric treatments for everyone, voluntary or not. They portray psychiatrists as money-hungry powermongers who push toxic medications
on people to further the interests of the pharmaceutical companies, and

they may see medication as the cause of symptoms rather than as a means to recovery. Why would anyone want what psychiatrists have to offer? Listening to these voices, it is hard to imagine that there are many people who benefit from psychiatric treatments and that there are many psychiatrists who find their work to be immensely rewarding. Activists often don't acknowledge that psychiatric symptoms really can render people dangerous or unable to negotiate their lives, and they see decisions to live on the streets or to cycle in and out of institutions as a "choice" without acknowledging that severe mental illness might alter the decision-making process. They also don't acknowledge that the civil rights of an individual may be at odds with the heartbreak of a caring family and that the concerns of loved ones cannot simply be ignored.

On the other side of the battleground are groups that push for the increased use of involuntary treatments. They are quick to point out that people with psychiatric illnesses often don't recognize that they are ill. From their perspective, this makes any concern about civil rights moot. In these discussions, treatment is often synonymous with medications, but they omit the downsides of psychiatric medications. Medications may cause some (but not all) people to feel sedated and slow, make them fat, destroy their sex lives, and increase their risk of getting heart disease and diabetes—problems that have the potential to decrease both the quality and the quantity of life. And the proponents of involuntary treatment don't acknowledge that patients, even after their symptoms have abated, are sometimes unhappy that treatment was inflicted on them. These patients are viewed as having no insight, are deemed the sickest of the sick, and treatment is forced for their own good, based on a doctor-knows-best mentality.

We join the battle with this book and advocate for the *judicious* and *limited* use of involuntary and humane psychiatric care, as a last resort, after every attempt has been made to thoughtfully engage patients in accessible, kind, and comprehensive services on a voluntary basis. That sounds like common sense, right? But oddly enough, in a world where mental illness has come to be equated with mass murder and escalating suicide rates, there is no place for common sense, and American society risks falling prey to a "round 'em up" mentality. When you get down to it, engaging reluctant people to get help can be costly and a lot of work. Why bother putting in all that effort to convince unwilling people to get care if you can simply force them? We have gone to great lengths to present a balanced view of involuntary treatment and all that goes with it, but we are not unbiased. Forced care comes at a cost, and it should be avoided except when it is the *only* way to get treatment for a person who is dangerous or tormented.

Federal and state legislation is often colored by fear. It is driven by legislators who want to say they are doing *something* to prevent mass murders. The National Rifle Association wants to be absolutely certain you understand: it's not guns that kill people, it's crazy people. Policy is now guided by emotion and reaction. It is no longer about creating realistic ways of keeping people safe and healthy in a nation that is hesitant to use its financial resources to help those who can benefit from services. At its heart, involuntary psychiatric care is a conflict among the desire of a family to care for a loved one, the need of a society to feel safe from real or perceived danger, an individual's civil liberties, and the imperative of psychiatry to respect patient autonomy while abiding by professional ethics.

These issues are complex and nuanced, and they can also be tedious. As in any political debate, each side cites the research that furthers its cause, and few people want to read a book of research studies. While we do present the research, we illustrate the issues by telling the stories of people who are involved with many facets of involuntary psychiatric care. Stories leave impressions in our mind and bring facts to life. This is the first time anyone has put the conflicting stakeholders together in the same book.

We'd like to take a moment to clarify some of the terms used throughout this book. At times we use the terms "civil commitment" and "involuntary hospitalization" interchangeably to refer to treatment in a hospital that is mandated by a legal process, against a patient's wishes. They are not always the same. Patients can be involuntarily hospitalized, then decide to become voluntary patients, or they may be released at a hearing. "Civil commitment" indicates that the hospitalization continues after a hearing on the issue. When it is necessary to make the distinction, we do.

The term "civil" indicates that these patients have committed no crime; their treatment is mandated to protect them or to protect members of society from the possibility that the patients' mental illness will lead them to do harm. Because the commitment is legally ordered, these patients do not have the right to leave the hospital, and they may consider their treatment to be forced. Each state differs in terms of how long a civil commitment can last without another hearing, and commitment often ends when the treating psychiatrist decides that the patient is well enough to be released. In other areas of medicine, patients can be treated against their will only when they have been deemed incompetent to make decisions for themselves because they cannot understand the treatment options. Psychiatry is the only field where someone may understand what is being offered and still be denied the right to refuse treatment.

We have tried to limit the use of the term "force" (versus "involuntary") to instances where a patient is physically restrained, but this is a nuance of language that has different meanings to different people. To people being ordered to swallow medication, it may well feel like force if they know that the consequence of refusing will entail being held down and injected. We also discuss outpatient civil commitment, where patients are ordered by a judge to go to treatment and to take medications outside the confines of a hospital.

We are psychiatrists, but we approached this book as an endeavor in journalism. We hope, however, that our expertise and experience have added a layer of understanding that a lay journalist does not have. As psychiatrists, we were able to gain access to settings that typically do not allow visitors. And we are good at getting people to tell their stories; after all, that's part of a psychiatrist's job.

To produce this book, we divided the labor. Dinah Miller conducted the interviews and visited the settings. She is part of the story, and the first-person voice is hers, unless indicated otherwise. Annette Hanson wrote about the historical and legal perspectives of involuntary treatment and summarized the research. She also has a personal story in the chapter on the use of restraint and seclusion.

We looked for stories that illustrated the different aspects of involuntary treatment. When we discuss patients and their families, we do not use their real names. Identifying facts are simply omitted; other details have not been changed unless we specifically indicate that they were—for example, in the chapter on guns and mental illness, the location has been changed and details have been altered. In a few instances, we also use pseudonyms for the doctors. Some of the examples were obtained from published accounts. In these instances, we have not changed the names of the people or the facts of the cases. Any place in the book where it is not clearly stated that a name has been changed, that is the person's real name. When we discuss incidents of mass shootings, we refer to these events by location rather than by the name of the gunmen because we don't want to contribute to their notoriety.

Because we are interested in giving everyone a fair opportunity to express their beliefs, those who are quoted at length were given the option to read their statements and correct any inaccuracies. It is our hope to avoid misinterpretation and sensationalism and to present all viewpoints in a respectful manner. All opinions and suggestions in this book represent a consensus of the professional judgment of both authors.

One

THE PATIENTS

Forced treatment casts a long shadow. If you work in mental health care, think about that, next time you're considering using it.

—Tweeted by "Mental Health" (@Sectioned)

Eleanor and the Case against Involuntary Hospitalization

"I would rather die than go in again. I am not depressed, and my psychiatrist considers me normal, but I can't live through that again. The staff was abusive, demeaning, and dismissive. I felt in fear for my life. Any lack of cooperation was met with physical and chemical punishment. Several of the staff gave me the impression that I would never be released and would spend my lifetime forcibly retained and chemically blasted into oblivion."

I could feel Eleanor's (not her real name) distress as she talked about her experience of being committed to a psychiatric hospital. Years had passed, but she still felt injured by her 21-day hospitalization in a private psychiatric hospital in Northern California.

"I still can't tolerate being in a car with windows closed because of the time spent shut in the confinement room with the lights out and no air circulating into the room. After several hours, the tiny room runs short of oxygen, so I needed to lie on the floor with my lips next to the space under the door, trying to suck some air through the single crack. I was afraid I would die in there of suffocation. That ought to be illegal. Some of what was done to us should be illegal."

Violation is a feeling we heard echoed by many patients, although some observers might dismiss Eleanor's distress. After all, she did get better, and people don't suffocate in seclusion rooms. And some might contend that Eleanor's behavior gave the staff no choice but to hospitalize her and place her in a seclusion room. But psychiatric treatment should not be

about punishing someone who is too sick to be responsible for her behavior. Seclusion keeps everyone safe until the patient is in control, but it
shouldn't be used instead of hiring more staff when increased supervision
might substitute.

Even if there are reasons that Eleanor's experience had to play out as it
did, we'd like to suggest that if many people leave a psychiatric hospital
feeling violated and demeaned, there is a problem. This is true even if
there are no clear answers as to what could have been done differently
and even if the distress is not universal. Instead of blaming Eleanor for her
suffering or suggesting that it's a product of her mental illness or perhaps
of an overly sensitive nature, we consider that her treatment could have
been kinder.

How often do people leave the hospital feeling as distressed as Eleanor
does? Research doesn't tell us, and it should. It's striking that Eleanor
continued to be preoccupied with her suffering years after her hospitalization. And we know that she's not alone; many people feel violated by
involuntary treatments, and that sense of violation sometimes persists
long after a person becomes well.

Eleanor's experience as a hospitalized patient was a one-time event in
her life to date; she is not someone who has been in and out of institutions,
and she made a full recovery from the episode of mental illness that led to
her hospitalization. Prior to that one episode at the age of 54, Eleanor had
never taken a medication for a psychiatric disorder. She does not use illicit
drugs, drink excessively, or have a history of criminal or erratic behavior.
She is a talented woman, and over the course of decades, she has been an
educator, a scientist, an artist, an explorer, a musician, an athlete, and the
owner of a successful business. She has a graduate degree and professional
certifications, and her personality is marked by what she calls "grit"—the
ability to push herself to succeed when others might simply give up.

Many people approached us with their stories. They saw their hospitalizations as unjust—the result of miscommunications among inept professionals—even though their behaviors clearly would have provoked
the other people in their lives to worry. We found that the stories of
these incidents varied greatly, depending on who was doing the telling,
and sometimes family members provided details that patients omitted.
When people are in a heightened emotional state, they may forget the

things they said or did while they were sick, or they may normalize or minimize their dangerous or bizarre behaviors as natural responses to being provoked. They don't see how their own irritability or psychosis may have been perceived as frightening by others. Some people expressed outrage that a psychiatrist committed them following a suicide attempt or after suicidal threats, with the suggestion that professionals should have known they would not have acted further on these ideas.

Other patients agreed to voluntary admission only because they were threatened with commitment if they did not agree to sign in, so while they were technically "voluntary" patients, the admission was coerced. Although this may seem like a matter of semantics, there is a legal differentiation, and we include Eleanor's story because we want to document the experiences of a patient who went through the process of an initial involuntary certification—in some states this is called a "72-hour hold"— followed by a civil commitment judicial hearing that allowed for longer inpatient treatment.

Eleanor started by seeking voluntary care and then ended up on a hospital unit against her will. She knew that there was something wrong with her, and in retrospect she acknowledged how unusual some of her actions were.

With streaked, light hair and an animated, rounded face, Eleanor looked quite a bit younger than her age when I interviewed her. She wore no makeup, and her lifestyle included hiking and a vegan diet. Eleanor's outpatient psychiatrist, Dr. Charles Johnston, did not begin seeing her until several months after her hospitalization. He did not know her during her episode of mental illness, but he treated her for years after, and he was able to provide an evaluation of her personality. Johnston described Eleanor in striking terms: "She is a very kind woman. She is open, caring, free-spirited, intrepid, and quirky." If his admiration for her wasn't obvious enough, he put his emotions in clear terms: "I kind of adore her." When asked about Eleanor's diagnosis, Johnston, who had been practicing psychiatry for 42 years when we spoke, replied, "I'm antidiagnosis. I may be antipsychiatry as it's done today. I saw her as being quite healthy."

Eleanor had a difficult childhood. Her father drank and was both physically and emotionally abusive. Her mother, a college professor, was often preoccupied with her work. Eleanor described both parents as perfectionistic and demanding, sometimes violent, with little tolerance for frustration. "I thought I was the sane one, and they were the crazy ones, so I tried to fly under the radar," she said.

The year Eleanor got sick was particularly difficult for her family. Both parents were ill and required a great deal of care. Her sister, who lived near them, shouldered much of the burden, and Eleanor made frequent cross-country trips to help. Her mother had Alzheimer's disease, and her elderly father was in the final year of his life. She felt terribly guilty when he eventually had to be placed in a nursing home just weeks before he died.

To add to all the sadness, four days after Eleanor's father died, her beloved dog died. "He was my favorite dog ever. A Marley-type dog, intelligent, with a mind of his own and deeply interactive," Eleanor said. The losses piled up.

In early August, Eleanor made the trip to attend her father's memorial service. She recalled, "My sister wanted me to do the eulogy. He was a bastard, and there was this contradiction between what happened and what I said." The eulogy she delivered left her feeling untrue to herself, hypocritical, and she was beset by memories from an unhappy childhood. She returned home, distraught, to a mountain of work for her business.

"It was stressful, and I was awake 24 hours a day for a month. My brain was not working right, and I drank a lot of caffeine. A pot and a half of coffee and two liters of Diet Coke every day for the 10 days prior to going into the hospital, and also, I was dieting. And instead of sleeping, I took on more things, more projects at work."

Eleanor later clarified that she did get some sleep during this time, but it was spotty and restless, sometimes as little as two or three hours a night, and her sleeplessness went on for a couple of weeks, not a full month.

In late August, Eleanor assisted with a dog rescue effort to save a group of abused animals whose condition upset her greatly. Two days after that, she spent a long day working outside in 95-degree heat. She suspects that she didn't drink enough fluids and may have become dehydrated. When a job took more time than expected because the client arrived late, the two of them had a disagreement, and Eleanor lost her temper. "This was very unusual for me. I never, ever, showed anger at my clients, but I was almost beyond angry. I was enraged and could not contain it as I normally would have."

Eleanor's husband, Frank (not his real name), returned from a business trip and noticed right away that something was wrong.

"This was the first time I'd seen her anxious. There was a desperation. . . . It was maybe frantic, and she didn't seem in control of her life. It's hard to describe someone's demeanor. It was the look in her eyes. She was a totally different person, and she had great concerns that she wasn't feeling as vibrant as she usually felt."

On the morning of the last day in August, Eleanor tried to sleep, but she couldn't. Her husband was angry that she hadn't taken care of a matter with the Internal Revenue Service while he had been away, and his anger upset her more. Overall, Eleanor felt exquisitely irritable, fragile, and sensitive.

Eleanor was taking hormone replacement medications for an underactive thyroid. For problems associated with menopause, she had started a progesterone regimen almost two weeks earlier. She wondered if her problems were related to the hormones. She called her gynecologist, Dr. Ricki Pollycove, who told her to come right in. Once Eleanor arrived, Pollycove walked her to the Emergency Department.

"It was a very stirring experience for me," Pollycove recalled. "She was disorganized in her thoughts; she hadn't slept for two nights. She was desperate and scattered, and she had this crazed look in her eyes. Her glasses were filthy. It was the only time in my professional career that I've escorted someone to the emergency room."

At the time Pollycove thought Eleanor was having a nervous breakdown. She noted during our interview, "We can all go over the edge when it gets to be too much." Pollycove reported that Eleanor did not say anything that led the doctor to believe she was dangerous, either to herself or to anyone else, and Eleanor made no mention of being fearful that anyone was trying to harm her. Pollycove noted that in her practice she made a point of being attentive to mental health issues, and she routinely screened patients for mood disorders before prescribing progesterone therapy because it can cause depression, irritability, and mood swings. The doctor's attention to psychiatric issues was not completely academic: her own sister suffered from bipolar disorder and died of suicide by jumping off the Golden Gate Bridge. She listens to patients more closely than the typical gynecologist does and said, "I like to think of myself as a 'gynachiatrist.'"

Dr. Pollycove did not think Eleanor would be admitted to the hospital. "I thought she'd be seen by a member of the psychiatric team, get medicated, and go home." If things had gone smoothly, perhaps that is what would have happened.

Eleanor's story unfolds throughout this book. We're going to leave her for a bit and end this chapter with a question. When we, as psychiatrists, are faced with a decision about involuntary care, the mind-set is usually one of "better safe than sorry." If we're not sure if someone is a danger to themselves or others, we assume it's better to hospitalize them than to have something catastrophic happen, and certainly there are times when that's absolutely true. If you assume that there is no downside to forcing care, then you hospitalize a lot of people. But how often would it change our decision if we routinely started with the idea that mandating care could have a bad outcome? Perhaps it's a bad enough outcome if the patient is still dwelling on their subjective distress years after the fact. But perhaps it's an even worse outcome—one that did not befall Eleanor—if forced care leads a person to refuse or avoid treatment at a later time.

Generally, psychiatrists don't think of hospitalization as being a potentially traumatizing event; they think of hospitalization as a way of getting much-needed treatment. But what if we, as a society, did everything we could to avoid treating people involuntarily so fewer people were traumatized and more people might be amenable to getting voluntary psychiatric treatment? Could it be that forcing care at one moment in time actually makes people less safe in the future?

Most people—the authors of this book included—agree that there are times when there is no safer or more humane option than to involuntarily hospitalize people with mental illness, even if that involves force. But if we step back and say that involuntary treatment is something that should be prevented if at all possible, then we would be starting from a different square.

Lily and the Case for Civil Commitment

2

"Nine years ago, I was involuntarily committed," Lily (not her real name) said.

I was extremely paranoid and afraid that people were tracking me down and that they thought I was a serial killer. My life was disintegrating at that time. I was paranoid with my professors at grad school and getting lots of incompletes, and I was accusing people at my job of weird things and then calling the police on them. I was convinced my landlord was spying on me. It took me a long time—probably a couple of years—to get fully better. The involuntary hospitalization was what got me started down that road. It was a stopping point from the spiral of psychosis and dysfunction I was in, and it allowed me to realize that I was ill and to put my full focus on getting better. I don't think I would have been committed if I hadn't had a psychiatrist who was treating me and a family who cared about me. I consider myself pretty lucky even though the police came and brought me in. Nothing really stands out about the hospitalization itself. At the time, I was the most terrified I have ever been.

Eleanor's story represents one perspective on the battle over forced psychiatric care, but it's not the only one. Before continuing with Lily's story, however, it's important to say that there were many people who wanted to discuss how they'd been injured by involuntary psychiatric hospitalization. It was much harder to find someone who believed that he or she had been helped by it. An online request for positive stories was answered by only four patients, two of whom were in Australia and South Africa. There are organizations composed of people who assert they have been injured by psychiatric treatments, of civil rights activists who strive to protect the rights of those with mental illness, and of parents who long to get much-needed help for their children—even if it means forcing that care. Yet there is no organization of patients who say they were helped by involuntary care and strive to make it available for others.

Lily, like Eleanor, connected the beginning of her illness to her father's death. Aside from that, however, Lily's and Eleanor's stories could not be more different. Lily was in college when her father died, and she was 30 years younger than Eleanor when her psychiatric saga began. And the course of her chronic psychiatric disorder was much more typical than Eleanor's.

Lily is a gentle soul. She was in her mid-forties when we spoke, and she looked a bit younger than her age, with dark brown hair that fell to her shoulders. Her right cheek was punctuated by the best of dimples. She talked in a halting, careful manner, choosing each word with deliberation, and her voice was that of someone 20 years younger. The innocence in Lily's demeanor was a contrast to how difficult her life had been while she was recovering.

Because she worked full time and lived across the country from me, we arranged to meet by Skype in the evenings and on a Saturday. She was late to the Saturday meeting because she was delayed getting home from her volunteer work with a local charity.

Despite her grief over her father's death during her junior year in college, Lily graduated on time from a difficult and prestigious university. The following year she was hospitalized on a voluntary basis for an episode of severe depression.

From there, Lily's story includes a number of episodes of depression, as well as suicide attempts by overdose, trials of different medications, treatment with a number of psychiatrists, and a second voluntary hospitalization. At one point, she enrolled in a study funded by the Stanley Foundation Bipolar Network, which she described as a longitudinal study to assess mood. She participated for two years.

Things changed when Lily was in her mid-thirties and living in Ohio. She went to graduate school there and worked in an administrative position. She entered treatment at a clinic that was part of a teaching center, and she began seeing a psychiatric resident in training, Dr. Gray (not his real name), for psychotherapy and medication.

Ten years later, Gray still remembered Lily, though he had moved to another country and no longer had access to her chart. "She had some interpersonal problems, but they didn't seem huge. She was a good patient, and she came every week. We only had to follow the patients for a year, but I decided to keep working with her," he said. "She was anxious and had difficulty juggling the demands of school and work. And she never liked her job. But then she started to think people were stealing from her at work, and she couldn't get her schoolwork done."

Lily also reported that things were unraveling for her at this time. "I started thinking the person I worked for didn't like me—that she was persecuting me—and I became actively psychotic. I called the police and saw things as having connections to an overarching plot. I also thought my professor was in on a serial killer thing."

Lily now recognizes that she was psychotic. This word has a precise meaning to psychiatrists. People are psychotic if they have hallucinations or delusions, or if their thinking is consistently and remarkably disorganized. A person with psychosis is unable to perceive reality accurately, and psychosis is often distressing and disabling. It is a sign of severe mental illnesses, such as schizophrenia, and it may also be present in people who have bipolar disorder or severe forms of major depression.

"I was emotionally upset," Lily continued, "and I called Dr. Gray, and he said I should come to the hospital. I didn't go to the hospital, and Dr. Gray sent someone to my apartment to talk me into going."

In fact, Dr. Gray sent a crisis team. When Lily refused to speak with them, he sent the police.

I asked Gray if, as a resident in training, he had consulted with a supervisor or if he had any doubts. "No. I was a fourth-year resident, and we were used to managing the Emergency Department without supervision, and I thought she was extremely delusional. She hadn't done anything violent, but I thought she could be a danger."

Lily remembered little about her hospitalization, and her records offered only a few details about what transpired. In our interview, she mentioned that a building site was being excavated across from the hospital and that she believed they were looking for bones to prove she had murdered people.

Lily's brother, Joe (not his real name), is a mental health professional, and he has a welcoming style of interaction. He recalled the time before Lily's hospitalization as being difficult. "I was very relieved when my sister was hospitalized," he said. "Really, it was a huge sense of relief that she was going to be taken care of. From a distance it was incredibly frustrating, but it was also kind of confirming. I had been thinking, my gosh, can people not see this? She was psychotic and talking about connections between things, and she was unpredictable. I was worried about her unpredictability, and she'd had suicide attempts before."

As Lily talked about her episode of illness, she gave more detail. "There was also a sexual component. I believed they thought I had molested people. And it was during the time of the 17-year cicadas, so they were everywhere. It freaked me out. My roommate in the hospital was kind of bipolar, and she had been drawing cicadas, and that was somehow part of it."

Lily recalled that she took medications willingly and found it reassuring when the nurses told her she was delusional. It helped her to hear that people were not really trying to harm her.

Her medical records reveal otherwise, however. She refused medications at times, and at one point a nursing note reads, "States it is not legal to keep her here, attempted to go AWOL while out on smoke break. Trying all the doors and refused to come back on unit."

Dr. Gray visited Lily on the inpatient unit, but she was convinced he was from the FBI and was not a doctor. "I felt bad for her. She had very little support, and she obviously wasn't comfortable. I talked to the treatment team about her."

Lily's family traveled to visit her from out of state. They took her to her apartment on a day pass, but she got upset and had to return to the hospital.

Joe recalled that afternoon. "It was intense at her apartment. It was a mess. I had to make some phone calls for work, and my sister thought they were about her. Then she accused me of going through her garbage. She couldn't find something, so she said someone must have come in and moved it."

"I felt angry, and wrongfully accused," he continued. "It's one thing to deal with mental illness as a professional. It's a whole 'nother thing to have to deal with it in your family. It's really scary."

Lily mentioned that one of the nurses was "creepy," but generally she felt that she was treated well in the hospital. Joe confirmed that nothing he saw made him worry for his sister's safety. Nor was he worried that she was being overmedicated. "If anything, I wished they were more aggressive in their treatment. I didn't see her getting better, and they were going slowly with the medicine. I felt like it was a little passive."

During that hospitalization, Lily was diagnosed with schizoaffective disorder, and she was treated with two antipsychotic medications, Risperdal and Seroquel. She remained in the hospital for a month. When she was released, she left Ohio and moved back with her family for a year. She saw a psychiatrist and was able to get Social Security Disability Income (SSDI) payments to subsist on during that time. It can be difficult to qualify for disability benefits, and people who do so lose the benefits if they work more than a certain number of hours a week or earn above a set amount of money, which means there is a strong incentive to remain disabled indefinitely. Few people return to the workforce full time after receiving SSDI. Lily, however, received SSDI for a little less than a year and then was well enough to move to another part of the United States and to resume employment.

Lily's life has not gone as smoothly as might have been predicted when she entered college. She's had a total of four psychiatric hospitalizations and years of job instability, as well as significant periods of time devoted to recovery. She has purposely overdosed several times, both before and after that first hospitalization. But while her life did not follow the trajectory it was on when she entered college, it has not gone all badly either. In many ways, Lily is lucky to be alive. She works full time and supports herself and a pet; she volunteers for a charity; and she has good relationships with her family, with her friends, and with the professionals who treat her. At the time we spoke, she had not been in a hospital for years.

Lily, unlike Eleanor, is in favor of forced psychiatric hospitalization. "I don't know for sure if it's good for other people. I do think it's sad that so many people are walking around with no one to intervene—people who are severely psychotic and marginalized by their illnesses. It's a shame there is not a way to treat people. I received this treatment because I had people who cared about me. I have mixed feelings about it because I know it can be traumatic."

Both Eleanor and Lily recovered from the episodes of psychiatric illness that led to their civil commitments. Both continued to get treatment, as needed, with a psychiatrist. But Eleanor walked away from her involuntary hospitalization feeling angry and violated, while Lily walked away feeling fortunate that she had been offered help when she was too sick to know she needed it. Eleanor's story may be more typical: many people feel violated by involuntary care. And it may also be the case that those who feel they were helped are not as vocal as those who were traumatized. The people who were helped may go back to their jobs and their families without any need to dwell on what was a distressing time in their lives.

Mark Komrad, MD, the author of *You Need Help! A Step-by-Step Plan to Convince a Loved One to Get Counseling*, shared his insights on the variety of responses patients have to involuntary treatment.

> I have found that patient attitudes towards their experiences, in retrospect, are not so much related to the involuntary nature of the treatment. Rather, their feelings are more about the way in which the involuntary process was deployed. Those who were approached with respect, dignity, explanation, professional compassion, and decency from law enforcement officers were more likely to appreciate the efforts when they recovered. Also, the degree of recovery is a factor. The more a person is able to emerge from severe psychiatric symptoms thanks to the treatment, the more accepting, understanding, even grateful they tend to be about the involuntary nature of that treatment.

Dr. Paul Appelbaum is a past president of the American Psychiatric Association and a forensic psychiatrist at Columbia University. His research focuses on how legal and ethical rules affect medical practice and research, and his publications on the topics of forced care and violence are considered classics. Appelbaum speculated about why some people become active advocates opposing psychiatric treatment.

> I don't know that there's one answer. My theory is that there are probably multiple variables that go into that. People have terrible experiences, and they are certainly more likely to respond with advocacy after an awful experience than after a good one. Some people have high levels of denial about their illness or their need for treatment and are likely to be angry

when they're treated involuntarily. And then there are these personality characteristics that drive activism in the general population that are probably just as relevant for people with mental illness. To be put in a hospital and treated against your will, I don't think any of us would enjoy that, and when it happens in a less than respectful way, I'm sure that heightens the anger. If people are angry afterwards, that makes a certain amount of sense, even if they recognize that it was in the end beneficial. It may be that it's too much to expect that people will be happy when we override their will.

Don't forget Eleanor and Lily. We're going to leave them for now, but we return to their stories later.

Two

THE BATTLEGROUND

If this becomes about who wins we all have lost. . . . It will be the most vulnerable people who will find out that big people with big words can't even get along with each other let alone sit at the same table to solve anything.

If it is only to be shots from a circular firing squad does anyone really believe there is a victor? There are a lot of good ideas out there. A lot of things might actually make a difference. But there is an even better and bigger idea that I hope someone hears:

This is not about us. Check your egos at the door. We have a much higher purpose.

The first agreement is that we must find a way to agree. Without that, all else is nothing but noise. Just more noise.

—Larry Drain, Wellsphere blog

In Favor of Involuntary Treatments

There is one thing that all parties agree on: the mental health care system in the United States is broken. It simply does not serve all of the people who need to be served, and it certainly doesn't offer care in a timely, user-friendly way. Some people fall through the cracks because they can't negotiate the logistics of getting treatment, while others decide they simply don't need or want the help that is available, for any number of reasons.

When it comes to involuntary treatment, the landscape is a contentious battleground, one where the artillery is so loud that one side cannot hear what the other side has to say. We believe that all the parties involved have valid points to make and that polarizing these viewpoints will not lead to answers. With one more swing of the pendulum, we risk becoming a society that focuses our resources toward forced care at the expense of denying services to those who *want* what psychiatrists have to offer. It's a mess.

What follows is a tour of the "combatants" on both sides. Those interviewed have beliefs about involuntary treatment that are subscribed to by thousands of others. Their views are presented from their perspective, and we have made every effort to create a respectful portrayal of their ideologies. We don't address the validity of their arguments in terms of factual accuracy, but their viewpoints are provided as a platform on which to display the major areas of disagreement.

E. Fuller Torrey and the Treatment Advocacy Center

The Stanley Medical Research Institute is housed in a nondescript office building on Connecticut Avenue, just inside the Washington Beltway. I met with Dr. E. Fuller Torrey, the institute's founder and executive director. Torrey is a schizophrenia researcher who has worked at the National Institutes of Health and at St. Elizabeths Hospital in Washington, DC; he is also known for founding the Treatment Advocacy Center (TAC), a group devoted to removing barriers to care for those with serious psychiatric disorders.

In the battle over forced psychiatric care, Torrey dominates the field: he has unequivocally put forth his belief that some people with serious psychiatric illnesses should be forced to get treatment if they refuse voluntary care. The author of many books, including *Surviving Schizophrenia* and *The Insanity Offense: How America's Failure to Treat the Seriously Mentally Ill Endangers Its Citizens,* Torrey holds back little. People with psychiatric disorders, he asserts, often go untreated; they often don't recognize that they are ill and in need of care; and society has done them, and itself, a great disservice by allowing them to go untreated. He sees the barriers to care as the elimination of funding for public psychiatric hospitals and legislation that protects the rights of people with psychosis to refuse treatment. Torrey is the one the media call upon to discuss how bad outcomes—violent crimes in particular—are preventable. Torrey goes a step further than most proponents of involuntary treatment; he believes that a subset of people should be required to get psychiatric treatment even if they are not dangerous to themselves or others. Forcing treatment, he asserts, may decrease the number of psychiatric patients who end up in jails and prisons—often for minor, nonviolent offenses—and could prevent mass murders. While he clearly has many supporters—a speech he gave at the annual meeting of the American Psychiatric Association in 2014 was met with a standing ovation—these assertions place Torrey at one end of the spectrum when it comes to the range of beliefs people have about involuntary psychiatric treatment. Some see him as a hero, others as a villain, and even among psychiatrists, his views are considered controversial.

Dr. Torrey is a slim, mild-mannered gentleman in his mid-seventies. The walls of his office are covered with colorful artwork and posters. He has white hair and a neatly trimmed white beard and mustache. He was a gracious host, even though he knew that I did not share all his beliefs about involuntary care.

"I started the Treatment Advocacy Center 15 years ago specifically to deal with the issue of how we can help people who are not being helped now, especially those with chronic and severe mental illnesses, such as schizophrenia and bipolar disorder. We know, at any given time, about 50 percent of people with schizophrenia and bipolar disorder are not being treated. And by far the largest reason is that they don't think there is anything wrong with them. If there is nothing wrong with them, why *should* they be treated?"

Torrey relied heavily on a term that is a relatively new (and controversial) addition to the psychiatric lingo, "anosognosia." Originally used to describe a phenomenon observed in patients who had strokes and who were unaware of the deficits they had as a result of damage to their brains, the term was extended to people with psychiatric disorders by Xavier Amador, PhD, the director of psychology at the New York State Psychiatric Institute.

I called Amador, and he explained anosognosia further. "It was a term that was originally coined by [Joseph] Babinski, a neurologist. I used to work at Long Island Jewish Hospital with stroke patients who had frontal lobe lesions. When I started treating psychiatric patients, I saw similarities between how they experienced their problem and how the neurology patients experienced theirs. There's a lack of insight about the illness, an unawareness. For anosognosia, we have at least three dozen studies showing anosognosia has some neural substrate."

"Anosognosia is the critical factor here," Torrey asserted. "It separates involuntary treatment from being a civil rights issue and makes it a biological one. It obviously makes a difference in how you think about it. If you think about it like the lawyers, it's a civil rights issue, and they want nothing to do with anosognosia because that confuses things."

"Anosognosia is a difficult concept to understand," he continued, "because it's difficult to imagine that someone does not know that they're sick. Say you're seeing Mrs. Jones, who had a stroke and can't move her left leg, and she's college-educated and says there is nothing wrong with her leg. So you ask her to move it, and she says it's tired now, perhaps if you come back later. Some people with schizophrenia know they are sick early on, but then lose it. John Hinckley—the guy who shot President Reagan—wrote a letter early on to his parents saying there was something wrong with his brain, but he didn't know what. Later, he had total anosognosia. I know because I examined him a few times."

"The studies have shown that about 50 percent of people with schizophrenia," Torrey said, "and 40 percent of people with bipolar disorder—mostly bipolar with psychotic features, I suspect—have some degree of anosognosia, sometimes complete."

Torrey talked openly about his sister who suffered from schizophrenia. "She had anosognosia, but she took her medicine regularly because she learned that if she didn't, she ended up back in the hospital, and she didn't like being in the hospital. But if you asked if there was anything wrong with her, she'd say no. Not in a million years would she say something was wrong with her. But she was not a problem in terms of medication because she didn't like to be in the hospital—she was hospitalized almost 25 years continually—and she wanted to be in the community. If you asked her why she was in the hospital, she'd say, 'I don't know. I had a cold when I went into the hospital.'"

Not everyone with anosognosia refuses medication, Torrey conceded. Some people feel obligated to do what their doctor recommends, whether or not they believe they have an illness. Torrey noted that some people with anosognosia later regain awareness as the medications treat their psychosis, and he postulated a mechanism that might involve the repair of neural circuits.

Dr. Solomon H. Snyder is a professor of neuroscience, pharmacology, and psychiatry at Johns Hopkins Hospital. He is best known for advancing the field by using receptor binding to characterize the behavior of neurotransmitters in the brain, and for the discovery of opiate receptors in the brain. I approached him for an opinion of this construct of psychiatric anosognosia. Snyder said, "I'm no great authority. In my personal experience, a substantial number of psychiatric patients lack appreciation that they are disturbed and so merit the anosognosia designation. In that sense, they are similar to neurologic anosognomics. It would be tempting to speculate that similar brain dynamics underlie the problem in psychiatric as in neurologic victims. However, we know nothing of the fundamental neural dysfunction for either group of patients, so it all remains in the realm of conjecture."

In talking about legislation for involuntary treatment, Torrey explained, "Most people will agree on the necessity of treating people who are a danger to themselves or others. Many disagree on treating people who are 'in need of treatment.' I personally am inclined to give people who are not aware of their illness a shot at treatment and would hospitalize them at least briefly and involuntarily to give them an attempt at medication to see if it does improve things, to give them a choice, basically. Other people would not agree with that."

When I asked for some specifics of such a plan, Torrey replied, "I would think two to four weeks in a hospital is a reasonable trial."

St. Elizabeths Hospital was the first federally funded public psychiatric hospital in the United States. Located in the District of Columbia, it opened in 1855 as the Government Hospital for the Insane; at its peak occupancy, around 1950, the hospital housed 8,000 patients. Torrey served as a psychiatrist at St. Elizabeths from 1977 to 1986, and he talked about his work there with patients who suffered from schizophrenia.

"There was a subset who were grateful, and there was a subset who had complete anosognosia and felt it was the worst thing that had ever happened to them, and that probably I was in cahoots with the CIA or KGB or whoever was sending the voices into their heads. I'd say the majority of them were not traumatized that much by [being involuntarily hospitalized]. At least, that was my perception. I followed them as outpatients later on, so I got to know some of them very well over the years."

One concern brought up repeatedly by those who oppose the use of involuntary treatments is that people who need treatment might avoid contact with psychiatrists for fear of being forced into the hospital or forced to take medications.

"In terms of scaring people away from seeking care," Torrey said, "I've heard that many, many times, always citing the same data. There was a study looking at this in the early 1980s in California, and it was scientifically totally worthless. I don't think involuntary commitment scares people away in terms of somebody who has never been treated."

It's a different story, he noted, when it comes to people who have already been involuntarily hospitalized. "There are some people who avoid care, and these are the ones who are the most vocal now. Some of them were treated poorly by professionals or hospital personnel who were not well trained or sympathetic. Obviously, these people are likely to stay away from care as best they can, and understandably. We need much better oversight: unannounced inspection of the wards at any given time, review of all the involuntary treatment, and review of all the seclusion room use, which we started when I was at St. Elizabeths. We cut it down to a very small amount. Most seclusion room use could be avoided."

Fuller Torrey's views about involuntary treatment come with a sense of optimism. He believes that forcing people to get psychiatric treatment—specifically, medications—offers the hope that people with severe psychotic illnesses might be able to negotiate better, safer lives, and he believes that such treatment could make a significant dent in the problems of homelessness, incarceration, and violence.

Ronald Honberg and the National Alliance on Mental Illness

The National Alliance on Mental Illness has traditionally been the group with views that are closest to those of Torrey and the Treatment Advocacy Center. NAMI was founded in the 1970s as a grassroots organization with local branches started by the parents of people who had schizophrenia. In those years, the "schizophrenogenic mother" was often blamed for her child's mental illness. NAMI became involved in education and worked to separate families from blame. The first national convention was held in 1979, and the organization now has a wide reach, with more than 1,100 local chapters and approximately 180,000 dues-paying members. NAMI states that one in four Americans suffers from a mental illness, and it no longer represents only parents or only patients with *severe* mental illnesses. In fact, the group could be said to have an identity crisis—it's not quite clear anymore exactly who it represents. Some people feel that the needs of those with severe mental illnesses—a very small percentage of Americans—are different from the needs of those who are able, as Freud said, "to work and to love" independently, without the need for hospitalizations or for high-cost, intensive services. But NAMI now lumps every executive who takes medication for anxiety together with those whose illnesses leave them homeless on the street.

When I approached a leader at a local NAMI chapter to ask for help in locating families to interview for this book, I was told that the group wouldn't help me. The topic was "too sensitive," and I was told that Dr.

Torrey could explain NAMI's views to me. That may have been the case for that one leader's views, but TAC and NAMI no longer see eye to eye on every issue. Torrey noted:

> I'm a member of NAMI. I've been a member since 1970 when it started, and I donated the royalties from the first edition of my book *Surviving Schizophrenia* to NAMI. I was active with NAMI through the late 1990s, and I gave talks at their annual conventions. Now, I pay my $35 a year in dues and criticize them frequently. I think the national NAMI totally sold out to the drug industry, which I think led it to have limited credibility. For the state NAMIs, at least half of them have totally sold out to the states, including Maryland, where the majority of their funds come from the state Department of Mental Health. In New York state, 92 percent of NAMI funds come from the state Department of Health. So they basically became a voice for the state. When the state Department of Health needs someone to go in front of the legislature and say how important what they are doing is, they simply have to pick up the phone and call NAMI to testify.

Torrey does approve of some of NAMI's activities. "At the local level, NAMI still does a lot of education. The family-to-family program is the core of NAMI, and a lot of family members learn a great deal about the illness of their family member this way. But NAMI's identity started out with severe mental illness, and now they have taken on all mental illnesses. They tried to become broader and very inclusive, and they let a small group of self-appointed consumer czars take over."

Torrey explained that a "consumer czar" assumes that everybody is alike regarding their awareness of illness and ignores the fact that some people are so ill that they become homeless or incarcerated.

Ronald Honberg is the national director of policy and legal affairs at the national NAMI office in Arlington, Virginia. Honberg lacks the intensity of the other activists I met with. He is a softer soul who was easy to connect with; he's as much about the encounter as he is about the mission. He started his career as a social worker; he had become interested in the field after having some difficult times as a teenager. He'd gotten treatment back then—treatment he'd found helpful—and did not go on to have a chronic psychiatric problem.

"I entered my own adult years with a sensitivity to the impact that mental health issues can have on young people, including stigma and the trauma of feeling that maybe my life was going to be derailed. That was part of it, but I also grew up in the sixties and seventies, and I bought into the mentality that we were going to change the world. I didn't see myself working for corporate America."

Honberg worked as a vocational rehabilitation counselor and then ran a group home before going to law school at night. When we spoke, he had worked at NAMI for 25 years. He started as a legislative advocate: "I didn't even know how to get to Capitol Hill at the time, let alone what to do when I got there."

Back then, NAMI had 7 employees. It has since grown to include more than 70. For the past 10 years, Honberg has worked with the board of directors writing policy positions, has written testimony, and has communicated with the media and state offices regarding legislation. He also does some lobbying, and his staff looks at issues in the military, in veterans' programs, and in child and adolescent services.

When it comes to involuntary treatment, Honberg—like many of the other mental health professionals I spoke with—asked me not to refer to it as "forced care." The NAMI website states clearly that involuntary treatment should be a method of "last resort." Despite that declaration, NAMI has traditionally favored legislation that would broaden the criteria that allow people to be brought in by the police for evaluations to include not only people who are dangerous but those who are gravely disabled—a broadly defined term that means someone is too ill to care for themselves—or even just "in need of treatment." In addition, NAMI has supported legislation to allow courts to order people to involuntary treatment as outpatients, a topic we look at in some detail in chapter 15. NAMI has also supported legislation that would permit mental health providers to share information with parents and caretakers, even against the wishes of patients.

My own interpretation of the NAMI mantra has been "take your medicines," and I shared that impression with Honberg. The organization holds the view that it's important to follow the wisdom of conventional psychiatry and that for serious conditions, such as bipolar disorder and schizophrenia, medications are necessary for life. While it is true that many people—perhaps as high as 90 percent of patients—will relapse after stopping medications for psychosis, there are some people who are able to come off medications and either don't relapse or else find alternative forms of treatment that work for their needs. NAMI has been slow to entertain this possibility, but the truth is that psychiatry does not have the best of crystal balls; some people who've been told they have a poor prognosis end up doing just fine.

"There are some people who misrepresent our 'mantra' for their own purposes," Honberg said. "There are people who feel like NAMI has strayed from its roots and will say to you, 'Oh, NAMI's not interested in people with serious mental illness anymore,' and people who are on the other side of the debate will say, 'All NAMI wants to do is tie people up and hospitalize them and forcibly medicate them.' And frankly, in my view, neither one of them is true. We're missing the boat when we argue that treatment is best if it's 'medical' versus 'recovery.'" Honberg continued:

> It's both, and 20 or 25 years ago we were a little myopic—and it wasn't deliberate, it's because that's what we knew and what we were told. The reality is that severe symptoms get stabilized with medication, and certainly we think medications need to be part of the treatment for most individuals. Not for all, and maybe not for their whole lives, and maybe not at high dosages, but they are a critical component of treatment. We also recognize that it's just a starting point of treatment, and you have to pay attention to the issues that matter to all of us—hope, work, and romantic relationships. I think there were a lot of psychiatrists who always felt that as long as we could get this person to take their medication, everything is just fine, and so what if their life is shit! We've evolved to realize that having a serious mental illness doesn't have to be a life sentence to misery. We didn't do enough 25 years ago to engender any hope.

As part of this shift, one of the speakers at the 2013 national NAMI convention was Robert Whitaker, a journalist who has asserted that psychiatric medications *cause* mental illness. In his book *Anatomy of an Epidemic*, Whitaker contends that as the use of psychotropic medicines has increased, so have the numbers of Americans who receive federal disability payments for mental illness. The pharmaceuticals, he says, sensitize a person's brain, leading to a worse long-term prognosis. Whitaker has started his own antimedication movement at a website called Mad in America, named after one of his books. The decision to invite Whitaker to speak at the NAMI convention was a controversial one that Honberg did not initially embrace.

Pete Earley, the author of *Crazy: A Father's Search through America's Mental Health Madness*, titled a blog post "Whitaker: Has NAMI Opened a Pandora's Box?" Earley wrote, "Did NAMI act irresponsibly giving Whitaker unmerited credibility when it asked him to speak or did it provide its members with a much needed different point of view?"

Since NAMI and TAC started in the same camp, and since I'd asked Torrey about his relationship with NAMI, I asked Honberg about NAMI's relationship with Torrey. He became uncomfortable and said he didn't want to discuss it. "It's adding flames to the fire." On the other hand, when the topic was Honberg's personal feelings toward Torrey, his affection and respect were obvious.

> I've never met anyone who cares more about people with serious mental illness than Fuller Torrey. He had as much to do with starting NAMI as anyone. If we had anyone on staff who was having a relapse—we've always employed a lot of people with lived experiences—I could pick up the phone and call Fuller and he would drop what he was doing. He'd come over to the office if necessary. He'd return calls from families at three in the morning. It really bothers the heck out of me personally—and this is me personally—that he gets vilified. I think he's frustrated at the lack of progress and barriers to getting people treatment. We continue to have members who have immense respect for Fuller Torrey and will tell you that reading his book *Surviving Schizophrenia* may have saved their lives and their marriages.

When it came to the topic of involuntary treatment, Honberg referred to this as "the nitty gritty": "We believe that if we had a really good mental health system, characterized by early identification and strategies to keep people engaged, more use of ACT [assertive community treatment] teams, more supported housing, and all the critical elements needed to achieve therapeutic gains and recovery, we would have far less of a need for involuntary treatment."

"We also recognize that there's a relatively small group of people, particularly when they get symptomatic, who don't have insight into the fact that they are ill and need help, and it's difficult to get them engaged. So we do believe that involuntary treatment as a last resort should be available," Honberg said.

"Our concern is that you never have any earlier resorts. People can't get services until they reach a crisis level, and at that point the only option that's considered is involuntary treatment. We have a job to promote better services for people, yet all the incentives are there *not* to treat people. The thing that troubles me is that once again we're getting completely fractured as a field. We waste too much energy arguing over things we can't seem to agree on."

Paul Summergrad and the American Psychiatric Association

While some people may assume that psychiatrists, on principle, are interested in forcing patients into care, the American Psychiatric Association (APA) has historically taken no formal position on involuntary treatment. All psychiatrists are bound by their own ethical judgment and by the laws of their state with regard to the emergency confinement of patients for evaluation and treatment. The APA is the largest body of organized psychiatry in the United States. While there has not been a formal stance on involuntary care, in 2015 the board of trustees voted to support federal legislation that included incentives for states to broaden the use of involuntary treatment, and in December the Board of Trustees of the APA took an official stance in support of outpatient commitment.

In the 1980s, the APA stood at the front line of the tension between those who wanted to liberalize involuntary care and those who opposed it. The arguments centered around the legal procedures and standards to admit patients involuntarily and to give them medication against their will. Proponents of treatment, including the APA, wanted a single legal hearing to permit both involuntary admission and involuntary medication, and they argued that the standard should be based on a patient's dangerousness.

The alternative view, proposed by those against involuntary treatment, is known as a "capacity-based standard." This standard is based on the belief that a patient's need for involuntary hospitalization does not mean that the patient is automatically unable to make decisions about treatment, specifically medication. Under this system, there are two hearings—one for involuntary admission and one for involuntary medication—each requiring a doctor to testify about the patient's symptoms and impairment.

The problem with a capacity-based standard is that it creates a risk that patients could be kept in the hospital indefinitely because they are unsafe for discharge, but also can't be given medication to reduce their symptoms and make them safer. In chapter 13, we discuss how a case in Maryland—and the legislation that followed—created exactly that situation. Another problem is that a capacity-based civil commitment law could allow ill people the freedom to hurt themselves or others.

"One of the implications of a capacity-based commitment standard is that a certain number of such people would be found to have capacity and could presumably then take their own lives," said forensic psychiatrist and former APA president Dr. Paul Appelbaum. In other words, if patients have the capacity to understand that they are suffering from the mental illness of major depression, and still want to commit suicide, they could be both competent and dangerous. "In these circumstances, [they] could not be detained for treatment."

While the APA considered the use of capacity-based treatment laws, it didn't go far with the idea for a number of reasons. Most psychiatrists are comfortable with the standard for commitment being "dangerousness" rather than "competence," and the APA looked at this after the states had already legislated their standards. Appelbaum concluded, "There was limited appetite for further tinkering, much less a reorientation of the approach to commitment."

I met Dr. Paul Summergrad in June 2014, a month after he was inducted as the president of the APA. We met at Tufts Medical Center, where Summergrad is the chair of psychiatry. He is comfortable wearing many different hats, and comfortable wearing them all simultaneously. He completed residencies in both internal medicine and psychiatry, as well as further training in psychoanalysis. He has certification in two psychiatric subspecialties, and besides being president of the APA and the psychiatrist in chief at Tufts, he served as the interim CEO and president of the Tufts Medical Center Physicians Organization.

Summergrad is an extroverted, approachable bear of a man. When we entered a restaurant, Summergrad excused himself for a moment to say hello to a group of Buddhists who were having a lunch meeting. He'd never met them before, but he explained, "I spent four years studying Zen Buddhism when I was between the ages of 19 and 23. At the end of it, I discovered I was a Jewish kid from New York who wanted to be a psychiatrist. I thought it was a transformative experience, and I'm sure there were people in my family who thought I could have benefited from psychiatric care at the time, but I wanted to take my own path. It's why I understand the importance of autonomy."

Summergrad set one nonnegotiable condition before he would allow me to interview him. While I wanted his input as the president of the American Psychiatric Association, which represents the interests of more than 35,000 psychiatrists, he was uncomfortable and unwilling to speak for the organization, but he agreed to talk about his own opinions.

"I think it's important for the APA to have a level of precision in [its] communications. Speaking personally, I think this is a very, very difficult set of issues. The APA doesn't have opinions—its board writes policy—but the APA is a membership organization, and its policies need to reflect the considered formal processes of the APA."

Summergrad continued, "I think people are divided about involuntary treatment, but I don't get a lot of email about this, and I don't know if they're divided 60–40, or 80–20, or 70–30." He was referring to the fact that there are no statistics on psychiatrists' attitudes toward involuntary care.

I think we've gone too far towards a standard of "imminent dangerousness" for commitment, and we need to move a little bit back towards "treatment," but I don't know where that dividing line is. Here's the way I think about it: if you bring together people who are reasonably fair-minded about this, there are some situations where everyone would say, "They're not behaving well, but it's their lives and it's their autonomy." In these cases, there shouldn't be any intervention from a legal or governmental perspective. If someone wants to live their life in a way that's stupid, or associated with some realm of stress or psychiatric illness, but they're not incompetent or close to being incompetent, I'm very sympathetic. On the other hand, there are situations where most people of good will, seeing the same thing that you or I would see, would clearly say, "This person's deteriorating and needs immediate medical intervention," and they should have that intervention. As a doctor who has to be on call, it affects me all the time. It's tragic to watch young people—and it's almost always young people—who have serious psychiatric illness where almost anyone would recognize they need care. Their parents, if they're in the picture, are desperately worried about them. But it's not until they reach the point of an imminently dangerous standard to themselves or others, or an inability to care for themselves in a community setting, that they can be hospitalized, and then if they pull together in a few days, we can't keep them. It doesn't make sense to me, because we know that they have an illness—one that puts them at long-term risk, including potentially significant and perhaps permanent brain changes—and we have treatment available. You can see a young person with bipolar illness walking shoeless in the Boston Commons, and you know when he's on his lithium he has a 4.0 GPA. It's heartbreaking, and his parents are desperately worried. Can you imagine being a parent in that situation?

We talked about whether psychiatrists might be motivated to want a looser standard for involuntary treatments either to increase their caseloads and incomes or to further the interests of the pharmaceutical companies. These are sentiments asserted by those who oppose current psychiatric practices.

"No," Summergrad responded emphatically. "Psychiatrists are overwhelmed by the number of people they take care of now. I don't think that enters into people's thinking."

He concluded, "I think the principle here is that no single person and no single group speaks for everybody. There are just too many types of illnesses subsumed here, too many points of view, and I think we need a really, really sober discussion about these very complex issues."

While Summergrad was not speaking as the voice of the American Psychiatric Association, his perspective was similar to those of many psychiatrists we spoke with. From a psychiatrist's point of view, psychiatric care is a good thing that helps people get better, especially when patients are tormented by voices, suffer from persecutory delusions, or are impaired by the misery of depression or the chaos of mania. Many psychiatrists, particularly those working in emergency settings, would like more leeway to determine who needs involuntary treatment when it comes to patients who are in desperate circumstances. Patients who are very ill may not be able to articulate that they feel violated by involuntary treatment. Meanwhile, those who treat them may see the situation as urgent, dangerous, and with little room for gentle care or calculated negotiation. A psychiatrist who treats patients in an emergency room or on an inpatient unit may have no idea that those treated forcibly have left feeling so terribly injured. Similarly, some patients who feel violated have difficulty appreciating that other patients find psychiatric treatments useful and that medications allow many people to live productive lives. Patients who feel violated may not appreciate that medication is life-saving for some. What we have learned is that in psychiatry, there is no room for a one-size-fits-all approach.

In many ways, those engaged on this battlefield seem to use the same rhetoric: involuntary care as a last resort, when all else fails, for the few patients for whom there are no other options, when the need for safety is paramount. As we hear in Eleanor's story, the lines are not always so clear, and as we hear from Lily, involuntary care may indeed be helpful.

4 | Against Involuntary Treatments

Having talked about groups that favor broadening the legal criteria to allow for more liberal use of involuntary psychiatric treatments, we now turn to those that oppose involuntary care. These groups have a wider range of beliefs. Some are opposed to using psychiatric treatments for anyone, even those who want what we have to offer. Others are less ardently opposed to all involuntary care, but their groups have historically opposed legislation that decreases patient autonomy.

Citizens Commission on Human Rights

Unlike the Stanley Medical Research Institute, the Church of Scientology in New York City is far from nondescript. The organization occupies a seven-story building in the heart of the theater district: on 46th Street, right off Broadway. A sign outside the imposing building advertised free personality and IQ testing, and although I had no appointment, the receptionist was gracious and called a gentleman from an upstairs office to come talk with me. She sat with me and waited until he came down.

Bob asked that I not use his real name and not record our conversation. He wore a business suit and conducted himself in a professional and formal manner, but he was clearly out of his comfort zone talking with a psychiatrist. Bob had discovered Scientology when he saw a commercial advertising a Scientology book on television. That was more than 20 years ago.

"They claimed to have the answers to life's more complicated problems. I thought they had a lot of nerve and that it was an outrageous idea that they had these answers, but then I read the book," he said, pointing to a display of *Dianetics: The Modern Science of Mental Health* by L. Ron Hubbard. I did not inquire into exactly what Bob meant by "life's more complicated problems," and I have not read the book.

Bob was working in New York City that week to help set up a free Scientology attraction, "The Touring Exhibit about Psychiatry: Help or Harm?" which both he and the receptionist invited me to attend. Just a few days earlier, there had been a Scientology protest outside the Jacob Javits Convention Center, where the American Psychiatric Association's annual meeting was being held.

In 1969 Dr. Thomas Szasz, a psychiatrist, joined with the Church of Scientology to found a mental health watchdog group, the Citizens Commission on Human Rights. The CCHR website states, "Psychiatric drugs cause: worsening depression, mania, psychosis, homicide, suicide, death. We believe involuntary commitment violates every fundamental human right."

Szasz, a professor emeritus of psychiatry at the State University of New York's Health Science Center in Syracuse, was best known for his 1961 book, *The Myth of Mental Illness*. He devoted his career to challenging mainstream psychiatry's reliance on diagnosis and medication. He died in 2012, and in his last videotaped interview at the age of 89, he talked about a patient who was involuntarily hospitalized.

"He was imprisoned. Let's call a spade a spade. He couldn't leave," Szasz said. He went on to talk about forcing patients to take medications, "which they call treatment, which I don't call treatment if you don't want something. If you don't want something, then in basic ordinary law, it's called torture."

On the battleground, the CCHR and the Church of Scientology represent an extreme viewpoint. They don't believe in the existence of mental illness, so according to them, there is no rationale for involuntary treatment under any circumstance. The CCHR public advocacy director had already told me via email that he could not speak with me, and he had directed me to the organization's website for information about its philosophy. I was pleased that Bob was willing to speak with me at all, even if he was a bit hesitant. Scientologists don't just oppose involuntary treatment, they oppose psychiatric medications in any situation.

"The subject is a fake subject. It's not the right solution to the problem,"

Bob said. "Psychiatry doesn't acknowledge the soul. It treats problems with chemicals." Despite this perspective, he told me that members were not forbidden from taking psychotropic medications or from seeking the services of psychiatrists. Yet when I asked how Scientology would respond to someone who takes a medication and feels better, he answered, "If they use cocaine, they feel better for a while too."

Bob had similar thoughts about involuntary care. "There are other solutions. When you understand why a person would behave irrationally, it's not a situation to be resolved by putting them on a hold [an involuntary observation period in a hospital], or on psychotropics, or in seclusion."

My discussion with Bob was brief. He gave me his email address but did not respond when I later tried to contact him. He left me with a postcard about the exhibit, some written material, and two DVDs: *Psychiatry: An Industry of Death* and *The Marketing of Madness: Are We All Insane?* The CCHR and the Scientologists represent an extreme antipsychiatry position, and it's important to note that their opposition to the field of psychiatry is based on an ideology.

Celia Brown, Janet Foner, and MindFreedom International

Unlike the Church of Scientology, other groups have come together around past encounters with the mental health system. Members of MindFreedom International refer to themselves as psychiatric survivors. Many have had side effects from psychiatric medications, which they believe were either prescribed unnecessarily, dosed too high, or prescribed in an irresponsible manner. In addition, many survivors have experienced involuntary treatments and a sense of powerlessness, and many feel that being given a psychiatric diagnosis, in and of itself, has been damaging to their lives. I found it interesting that several people involved with the mainstream psychiatric community suggested that I should not include the perspective of either the CCHR or MindFreedom International in this book.

The website of MindFreedom International describes the organization as a "nonprofit organization that unites sponsor and affiliate grassroots groups with thousands of individual members to win human rights and alternatives for people labeled with psychiatric disabilities."

The group was founded in 1986 by Harvard graduate David W. Oaks.

Oaks had been repeatedly hospitalized at McLean Hospital, a Harvard teaching hospital, during his undergraduate years in the 1970s. His treatment included forced medications and seclusion. After discharge from the hospital, he did a student project with a survivor group, the Mental Patients Liberation Front. Oaks graduated from Harvard with honors and later started his own movement, modeled on the civil rights movement. In 2005, the group adopted its current name, MindFreedom International, and Oaks served as its executive director until 2012, when a tragic accident left him disabled. In a 2010 YouTube video, he gave a tour of the MindFreedom office in Eugene, Oregon—including a quick hello from his 93-year-old mother, who volunteered for the organization. Oaks noted that MindFreedom challenges the power of the drug industry, sponsors Mad Pride events, and promotes choice.

"Some of our members choose to take medicines, but we are willing to talk about the bully of drug company abuse. We're a nonviolent revolution in mental health," Oaks explains in the video.

Celia Brown is the president of the board of MindFreedom. When I initially contacted her, she was hesitant to talk with me. She worried that her words might be taken out of context or used to further the case for more forced care, and it troubled her that I had spoken with E. Fuller Torrey, whose mission directly counters those of patients' rights groups. Brown finally agreed to a conference call, which included Janet Foner, the executive director of MindFreedom.

Both women talked about the organization. Foner noted, "We have individual members, and there are over 100 groups around the world. They are made up of survivors as well as lawyers, family members, and doctors—anyone who wants to fight for human rights in the mental health system. I think we have 1,000 or more dues-paying members. But there are over 10,000 people on our email list. A lot of people can't afford dues; it's a poor people's movement." Brown told me a little about herself: in addition to being a psychiatric survivor, she had also survived trauma and breast cancer. At the time of her psychiatric hospitalization, she was given a poor prognosis and told she would not be able to accomplish much and would not have children, so she was particularly proud that her son had just graduated from high school. She has found tremendous support in the MindFreedom community.

"When I found the movement, I found myself. They supported me on my journey of recovery, and it was very healing. Activism and social change make people heal, it gets them energized. It's not treatment that saves the person from themselves, it's being around supportive people."

Like Brown, Foner is an avid activist. She is one of the founders of MindFreedom, has held several leadership roles in the organization, and has worked for the League of Women Voters. In addition, she has a leadership role in the Re-evaluation Counseling movement, a Seattle-based international organization that promotes peer co-counseling as a means of social change. At the time of our conversation, Foner had been married for 45 years; she has two adult sons.

In 1967, Foner was hospitalized for 10 months. In the first days of her hospitalization, she reported, she was injected with an antipsychotic medication, Thorazine, in high enough doses that she passed out, and she was placed in seclusion twice, for many hours. Although she described being dragged into the hospital by two attendants and a nurse without being told that she was being hospitalized or why, she did note that there were aspects to her care that were not completely negative.

"I was lucky I had a psychiatrist who was wonderful to me, and he helped me get off the drugs by gradually reducing them. I was on psychiatric drugs for a year and a half. A lot of people think that because I'm fighting for psychiatric rights that I must hate psychiatrists and I must have had a terrible time with mine, but I actually had two excellent psychiatrists who listened to me and were actually fine with me crying and things like that. I was lucky. That wasn't the case for a lot of the people I was in the hospital with."

Foner was hospitalized approximately 50 years ago, and many things have changed about involuntary treatment since then. There are now laws that regulate the use of seclusion and restraint and the administration of involuntary medications. The power of Foner's sense of violation, however, has been strong enough to drive her advocacy for decades.

Brown discussed what MindFreedom does:

> I would say we get 100 to 200 calls a month, generally from people who are tired of the treatment that they are getting, and they find MindFreedom on the web or someone tells them about it. They call and feel so welcome that they have found someplace where they can share what happened to them. We work with them and try to support them. First, we try to stop

the forced drugging or electroshock from happening. We have a volunteer list and MindFreedom Shield. The MindFreedom Shield is loosely based on the Urgent Action Network as run by Amnesty International in the sense that people act together in a nonviolent way to support the human rights of the person asking for assistance from us. The Shield gets activated, and we get volunteers who support the person on the inpatient unit. We will call the hospital, or if there is something else that person wants us to do, we do it. And a lot of times that will stop the force. It takes a lot of organizing and talking to the administrator of the hospital or sometimes the governor of the state or the commissioner of mental health.

"We have a lot of sponsored groups where we can link them up for support and where they can get alternatives," Brown continued. "We do have meetings. There are MindFreedom affiliates—I'd say we have about 20 affiliates, and we're getting more internationally. You know, the mental health laws do not support us, so we have to take human rights into our own hands in mental health."

While survivor groups are linked by a shared sense of victimization by the psychiatric treatment community, survivors are often people who have been able to function without a continued need for psychiatric medications and treatments. As part of their belief system, survivors object to the medical model of illness and treatment. They claim that psychiatry has overemphasized the scientific basis of its disorders and treatments by stating that medications correct a "chemical imbalance," even when the precise neurochemical cause for any specific disorder has not yet been elucidated.

It was clear from listening to Brown and Foner that they believe there are better ways to treat people diagnosed with psychiatric illnesses than what conventional psychiatry has to offer. They talked about using alternative treatments for psychosis that do not rely on medications. Still, the organization does not forbid its members from taking medication. Foner was quick to tell me that because MindFreedom does not believe that psychiatric illnesses exist in the medical sense, they do not like the term "medication" and prefer "psychiatric drugs."

We have a position that people have a choice as to whether or not they take psychiatric drugs, but many of us who are active in the organization agree that we're against psychiatric drugs, because we see the harm that they do. But we're not against the people who use them, and we don't tell people who want to take them that they shouldn't take them, because that's counterproductive. Somebody who's unhappy with the drug will figure that out, and somebody who likes it, maybe eventually they'll figure out how damaging these drugs are as well. However, if we tell them "you're terrible for taking the drug," that's not going to get anybody anywhere.

The MindFreedom leaders feel that compassion and human connection are instrumental means for treating mental illnesses, even for the most ill and violent of patients. When I asked Foner what might work better than traditional psychiatric treatments, she replied:

There's no black-and-white situation. People need emotional support, and they need to be able to release emotions. A lot of times — and this may go counter to what you've been taught in your training — people just need to cry, or they need to tremble or get upset and vent, and oftentimes if that were done without giving somebody psychiatric drugs, things would proceed in a lot better manner. But because there is a mind-set that someone is dangerous if they are having a lot of feelings or delusions or whatever, things can escalate. And if you give someone psychiatric drugs, it just complicates things way, way, way more because the person is upset and giving them psychiatric drugs keeps them from being able to cry and shake and rage, which is what they need to do in order to heal. A lot of times we talk about "what would you do instead?" Well, you'd go on a hike, or you'd go camp out in the woods, or you'd go be with friends. That kind of simple human situation is oftentimes much more healing than the conventional mental health system. So people are often treated with something that is counterproductive to what they really need.

I pushed a little more and asked what Foner thought should be done with very sick and violent patients, and whether forced medications are ever indicated.

First of all, there is a myth that mental patients are violent. If someone is violent, then I think you need someone who can handle that. I'm not speaking for MindFreedom here; this is my personal opinion. If someone is violent and they've committed a crime, then they should go to jail. But suppose they haven't committed a crime, but they are punching people. Then you need somebody who can do karate or aikido or somehow be able to protect themselves and yet get in there with the person and give them a punching bag and let them punch the punching bag. If the helper believes that the person is capable of releasing emotions, it will make a big difference. Sometimes people will get angry and start punching people. They need an opportunity to let go of their rage in a safe way, in a safe place, where they can't hurt anyone. You don't isolate or restrain someone or give them drugs. This just increases their anger.

Foner's perspective sounded idealistic, and I later found myself wondering about the logistics of such a plan. In the case of a violent psychotic person, what would happen if he or she couldn't be gently corralled into a room with a person skilled in martial arts? What would transpire if that person wasn't able to punch out their emotions on a punching bag?

Brown added, "I agree with Janet. We live in a violent society, and I think that people labeled with mental illness are the scapegoats. We do have alternatives that are not recognized or funded but really work for people." They specifically mentioned Open Dialogue, an alternative Finnish approach to addressing psychosis, and the Hearing Voices Network. "There are a couple of support groups in New York City and internationally, and people can go to a safe place and talk about what they are experiencing, but this is never thought of when people are acting out or violent. Instead, we restrain the person and give them drugs, and this is never helpful in the long run."

Both women expressed their belief that objections to psychiatric hospitalizations are universal among patients.

Foner noted, "Voluntary commitment in a mental hospital is pretty much a euphemism. In such cases, patients will often sign into the hospital, so the admission is technically 'voluntary,' but the patient is told that if they don't sign in, they will be committed. That was the case for me. I was voluntarily committed, but they told me if I didn't go in voluntarily, they would get my mother to commit me. It wasn't a choice."

We discussed the difference between people who refer to themselves as "survivors" and those who call themselves "consumers"—the group represented in the next section. Foner explained, "I would say the difference between psychiatric consumers and survivors is in name only.

Mental health consumer sounds like people *want* to consume mental health products, but when you talk to a mental health consumer for a long time, you find they are just as unhappy with treatment as survivors. Nobody really likes it that I know of."

While the MindFreedom leaders assert that psychiatric hospitalization is a bad thing, and they clearly oppose forced care, their beliefs about *voluntary* hospitalization do not fit with our clinical experiences. There are patients who feel distressed and desperate and who want the opportunity to be treated in an inpatient setting, and many are prevented from entering the hospital because of the lack of available beds, or because their insurers refuse to cover inpatient admission. Of those who have been admitted for voluntary care, many feel it was beneficial. The views of MindFreedom International remain clearly opposed to those of mainstream psychiatry.

Daniel Fisher and the National Empowerment Center

Severe psychiatric illnesses destroy lives; some diagnoses have become associated with poor prognoses. Some people with psychiatric illnesses, especially schizophrenia, are derailed from their personal and vocational goals, and psychiatrists traditionally have told these patients not to set their sights too high and to decrease stress. They may have encouraged patients to pursue disability benefits through Social Security, rather than to reenter school or the workforce. Severe psychiatric illnesses can be associated with a lack of hope.

One thing we've heard repeatedly, however, is that people don't like being told that a psychiatric disorder, no matter how severe, means they won't amount to much. The backlash to such a dismal, and sometimes unfounded, foretelling of the future has resulted in the recovery movement, which strives to empower patients and reclaim hope. While the recovery movement may include the survivors we discussed in the previous chapter, it also welcomes current patients, or consumers, as they prefer to be called. Those in the movement strive to maximize their social and occupational potential, and they may rail against the idea that certain psychiatric diagnoses doom people to a diminished life with a poor prognosis.

The term "recovery" speaks to maintaining consumers' autonomy and having them take a proactive role in their treatment with an emphasis on peer supports. The recovery movement, however, is not at odds with a medical model approach to psychiatric disorders, and in general patients are neither forced to take medications nor discouraged from doing so.

In 1968 Daniel Fisher had just finished graduate school and had begun working as a scientist at the National Institute of Mental Health, where he was doing schizophrenia research. When I interviewed him, he explained that he had worked with the Public Health Service as an alternative to entering another branch of the uniformed services during the Vietnam War. His research was going well when he became psychiatrically ill himself. Dr. Fisher was diagnosed with schizophrenia—the illness he studied—and was hospitalized three times between 1969 and 1974. He has not been hospitalized since then.

> The whole period is a little confusing. I was working as a neurochemist on dopamine and serotonin synthesis, and the work drove me crazy. The process of doing research drove me crazy because I was good enough as a biochemist, as my boss would say, that I really got into the problem. I actually believed I was the enzyme I was studying. I was terrified, and so I stopped working, and I felt there was no reason to go on moving, or living. From a psychiatric standpoint, I had catatonia, and I just stopped all activity. All they could do was take me to a hospital. I went to Bethesda Naval Hospital. In military hospitals, there are no commitment hearings; they just order you in. While there were some positives from being in the hospital, overall I was so furious at spending five months in that hospital.

In a speech he gave in front of the Boston State House in 2012, Fisher declared, "In my twenties I was psychiatrically hospitalized and locked in a solitary confinement room with no furniture. That was called 'therapeutic seclusion.' I was restrained and forcibly injected with mind-numbing drugs and that was called my 'therapeutic plan.' Years later I still carry the outrage of that torture as deep wounds in my soul."

Unlike most other activists, Fisher was determined to conduct his struggle from inside the profession. He already had a PhD, but while he was in the hospital, Fisher decided that he wanted to become a psychiatrist.

> I don't know if you can imagine what it's like to be locked up in a psychiatric hospital. Even if you're working there, it's hard to imagine what it's like not

to get to go home and not to know when you'll get out. All they'll say is terrible things like, "When you act appropriately, you can leave." There are no good explanations; it's not like there's a blood test or like your glucose has to reach a certain level. And then you get angry, and when you get angry you [get put] into seclusion. The reason I wanted to become a psychiatrist was to let people out of these hospitals or to create alternatives to hospitals.

Despite his distress in the hospital, Fisher told me about the kindness and flexibility of his psychiatrist and that he felt most helped by the corpsmen. "The corpsmen in the navy were the least trained. They were young kids—18 and 19 years old—with very little formal training, but with great instinct, and their instinct was to help. For one entire month I did not say a word, but I was watching, and what I was watching for was signs of human contact, and they established it."

Fisher graduated from the George Washington University medical school in 1976, then moved to Massachusetts to do his residency in psychiatry at Cambridge Hospital, a Harvard training program. His move to Boston was motivated by a desire to be involved in the Mental Patients Liberation Front, the same advocacy and support group that David Oaks, the founder of MindFreedom International, had been involved with. During this time, Fisher did not disclose to his colleagues in psychiatry that he had been diagnosed with schizophrenia.

In 1992 Fisher co-founded the National Empowerment Center. The NEC's mission, as stated on its website, is to carry a message of recovery, empowerment, hope, and healing to people with mental health issues, trauma, and/or extreme states. He noted that the members of the NEC want society to realize that people with mental illnesses are people first. "And that we're not all ax murderers."

Fisher also talked about a program he teaches called Emotional CPR: "It's a public health program for any person helping another person through an emotional crisis. C is for connecting, P is for empowering (mostly by equalizing the relationship by sharing something of your own emotions when you're with someone), and the R is for revitalizing, which is to bring back people's vitality. It just works like a charm; you'd be amazed."

We discussed what to do in situations where people may become violent or where hospitalization may be seen as unavoidable.

"You reach them before that. There are always antecedents. People don't just become violent out of nowhere. I worked for three years in a psychiatric hospital, and the only instances I saw of violence were when there was bad communication between the staff and the people receiving services, and when they were treated disrespectfully or were misunderstood. Of course, I think it's better not to hospitalize if at all possible. But I'm not someone who says there will never be any forced treatment. I just think we can scale it way back."

Daniel Fisher is a remarkable man with a remarkable story, and his experiences have given him a unique opportunity to know the worlds both of the psychotic patient who is at the mercy of a treatment team and of the physician who is struggling to help people in the throes of mental illness. He has written:

> For 35 years, I have provided psychiatric care to mental health consumers in hospitals and clinics, including many years as the medical director of a community mental health center. During this period, I have also been part of the consumer movement. The tension of seeing and feeling both of these often antagonistic sides of the system has been painful yet rewarding. By working intensely with providers, families, and consumers, I have learned to translate their worlds to each other. I have found that recovery is the common ground uniting these groups. To reach this common ground, psychiatrists had to stop believing that remission was the best anyone could hope for, and parents needed to understand the importance of their children gaining greater autonomy. Consumer leaders had to accept that there is something fitting the description of mental illness for which they need assistance.

While Fisher's viewpoint seems reasonable, some people feel that the recovery movement's mission is a misguided one. Liza Long is the parent of a child with mental illness, an advocate, and a writer. In an article in the *Huffington Post*, Long wrote that she wished the word "recovery" would not be used. She has contended that not everyone recovers, and the movement inadvertently blames and stigmatizes those with an illness who don't get better.

In many ways, the recovery movement has been successful in aligning itself with mainstream psychiatry. It's difficult to argue with hope and empowerment. Medicine, including most specialty fields, has come to embrace the inclusion of the patient as a partner in making health-care decisions, and psychiatry—for the most part—is no exception.

Ira Burnim and the Bazelon Center for Mental Health Law

Patients, survivors, and consumers have a vested and personal interest in matters regarding forced psychiatric care. Many of them, however, go through periods in the course of their mental illness when they are too compromised to advocate for themselves. There is another group of individuals that has a less personal, but no less passionate, stake in the outcome: civil rights attorneys.

Ira Burnim is the legal director at the Bazelon Center for Mental Health Law in Washington, DC. The Bazelon Center—originally called the Mental Health Law Project—was founded in 1972. Before we even met, Burnim was quick to tell me that he doesn't believe that involuntary treatment is the issue our resources should be focused on.

> We are concerned that forced treatment is increasingly perceived as a panacea for the ills of the mental health system. Our analysis—which as far as we can tell is widely shared by the leadership of public mental health systems and by the federal government—is that the primary problem with the public mental health system is that there is a severe shortage of voluntary services, such as assertive community treatment, intensive case management, mobile crisis services, supported housing, and supported employment. These services, with proven effectiveness in meeting the needs of individuals with serious mental illness, are greatly preferred to forced treatment, and do not have the "side effect" of driving individuals away from the mental health system.

The Bazelon Center was founded by a group of lawyers who brought the first big litigation in the disability rights area, *Wyatt v. Stickney*. The 1971 class action suit against Bryce Hospital in Alabama was a landmark case, the first to establish that involuntarily hospitalized patients had a right to treatment and that a court could establish specific requirements for constitutionally adequate care. Like many public interest organizations, the Bazelon Center started out as a litigation law firm, then expanded into policy advocacy and public education.

I met with Burnim in the Bazelon Center's twelfth-floor conference room. He's a talkative, intense, and passionate man. "A couple of years ago, when policy discussions were not framed by Newtown and gun violence," he noted, "the issues were more about how we could implement the vision of the Americans with Disabilities Act so that people with disabilities can live lives like people without disabilities."

Burnim talked about initiatives to provide housing for people with psychiatric disorders and to provide services for those with serious mental illnesses in ways that meet their needs. He is very much in favor of using assertive community treatment teams for those with persistent mental disorders. An ACT team is a multidisciplinary group of mental health professionals, including nurses, social workers, rehabilitation counselors, and psychiatrists, who provide assessment, treatment, and case management services. Services may be quite comprehensive and include supports critical to helping the individual manage in the community. ACT services are ideally available around the clock and on weekends, and ACT services are traditionally voluntary; the patient must agree to receive them. Some groups, however, see ACT teams as intrusive and even unwelcome, a way for psychiatry to exert a coercive force by coming to people's homes and helping them comply with treatment.

Burnim talked about the importance of providing housing to those with severe mental illnesses:

> Housing-first strategies work. You need to go out and ask people what they want, and how they want to change their lives, then help them do it. Those kind[s] of strategies have enormous success in keeping people in treatment. Traditionally, housing programs [were] linked to substance abuse treatment, and required people to abstain from substances use. Housing-first programs provide housing to people who may be actively drinking or using drugs.
>
> The people who commit crimes and end up in jail are primarily people who are homeless. We worked with the police over a period of years, in a number of locations, and they were pretty clear that they thought the best way of addressing the cycle of people going in and out of jail was to give

homeless people housing, and it turns out there's a lot of research that supports that. It's really hard to get better when you're homeless.

Burnim talked about the deinstitutionalization movement that started in the 1960s as the state psychiatric hospitals eliminated beds and released patients into communities. At their highest occupancy rate in the mid-1950s, state hospitals housed over half a million Americans. In 2010, only slightly more than 43,000 state hospital beds remained. While Fuller Torrey contended in his book *The Insanity Offense* that deinstitutionalization was the direct cause for increases in the number of people who are homeless and incarcerated, Burnim disagreed.

> This kind of narrative, that the homeless mentally ill happened as a result of deinstitutionalization, doesn't conform to the actual chronology. Homelessness in this country developed when the Reagan administration slashed federal housing programs, and [those programs have] never recovered. People know the narrative that when we deinstitutionalized, the money didn't go into community services; it disappeared. If you follow from 1955, at the height of the institutional population, forward, you see a decline in real dollars in mental health budgets, and so you had a massive disinvestment in mental health and housing support. Also, there were some economic changes in the real estate market—think about New York City—that eliminated what wasn't a wonderful option, but was at least an option that existed for a lot of poor people: SROs [single-room occupancies]. Times Square was full of those places, and they disappeared. It happened in a lot of other cities too.

The Treatment Advocacy Center has contended that there are not enough state hospital beds to meet society's needs. Torrey has asserted that a minimum acceptable number of state hospital beds would be 50 per 100,000 residents, but only one state, Mississippi, currently meets this minimum. Burnim disagreed with the idea that there are not enough hospital beds.

"Emergency Departments get backed up, but it's not the lack of hospital beds, it's the lack of community services. If you put all your money into hospital beds, you never stop the flow of people coming in. It's a vicious cycle."

Burnim also disagreed with Torrey's assertion that involuntary treatment makes society safer.

One of the biggest challenges is that the public fears people with mental illnesses. And the public will pay attention if we start scaring them. It's clear that is the reason Torrey's in the media all the time, while no one else in the mental health community is. It's because no one else has that compelling soap-opera story. TAC's method is to tell people there are all these folks who are out of their minds who may kill you, and the only way to stop this is to forcibly medicate them; that's the entirety of TAC's message. The public does not value people with serious mental illness or homeless mentally ill people. If they did, they might give them housing. It's just not a high enough priority.

Burnim went on to talk about the role of involuntary treatment in preventing violent tragedies. Most people, he noted, are involuntarily hospitalized because they present a danger to themselves.

How many people are actually being committed for being a danger to others? My experience is those people don't get out of the hospital, or they end up in jail or in state hospitals. This question always assumes that in the community there are no effective interventions for dealing with this, and that's not true. There may be some very small group of people who don't respond and remain dangerous, but this is a hypothetical question for books and TV shows. The people I know like this are all in institutions. And medicines don't prevent people from being dangerous—it's not like you give people medications and the problem is solved. At every level, violence and involuntary treatment are the issues dominating public discourse about mental health.

Burnim's view is that the current media frenzy to link violence and mental illness is detrimental to those with psychiatric illnesses.

"If people are dangerous, you can forcibly hospitalize them—that seems like a necessity—and we've never been against that. But I think it's quite discriminatory; it's always been true of civil commitment that the only people in the US who can be preventively detained are people with mental illness. If there's about to be a gang fight, but the gang members haven't done anything *yet*, you can't round them up and confine them because they're dangerous due to delinquent and violent tendencies. It's a historical artifact developed as part of our law."

Burnim concluded, "The thing we all agree on is that the current mental health system is a wreck, and—at best—it responds to people when they're deeply in crisis, and then usually in a coercive way."

Three

CIVIL RIGHTS

We hold these truths to be self-evident, that all men are created equal, that they are endowed by their Creator with certain unalienable Rights, that among these are Life, Liberty and the pursuit of Happiness.

—*Declaration of Independence*, July 4, 1776

Eleanor, Lily, and the Process of Civil Commitment

Eleanor went to the Emergency Department, and things didn't go smoothly. We'll talk about Eleanor's care in the ED in a later chapter, but for now we're going to skip ahead in her story to explain the legal process used to hospitalize her against her will and where this process came from.

After a long and disturbing day, Eleanor arrived in the ED screaming inconsolably. She was seen by a physician, who filed an application for a 72-hour detention for evaluation and treatment. He checked off a box indicating that Eleanor was a "gravely disabled adult" and jotted a three-line handwritten note indicating that Eleanor was agitated, that her thoughts jumped from one topic to another, and that she was paranoid. He wondered if she might be suicidal. He commented that there was no history of drug abuse, which could have provided an alternative explanation for Eleanor's symptoms. He then sent her by ambulance to a psychiatric unit several miles away.

Eleanor was admitted to the psychiatric unit on an involuntary 72-hour hold at 10:35 p.m. on September 1. She had gone to the ED for help and said she would have signed herself in for evaluation voluntarily, but that option was never offered. She arrived on the psychiatric unit tired and noted, "I was afraid to go to sleep. I was afraid they were trying to kill me."

Eleanor's 72-hour hold ended at 9:50 p.m. on September 4, but her doctor determined that she required further hospitalization. By California state law, a hearing was required to allow for up to two more weeks of involuntary hospitalization. From there, the process in California varies,

depending on whether patients have been deemed to be a danger to themselves, to be a danger to others, or to be "gravely disabled," as Eleanor was.

We don't know how often people are admitted involuntarily across
the United States. Dr. Brian Hepburn was the executive director of the
Department of Health and Mental Hygiene of Maryland when I communicated with him, and he was able to provide some statistics for his state.
To be "certified" in Maryland, two physicians or psychologists evaluate
the patient and determine that the criteria have been met for involuntary
inpatient care. In 2012, 6,889 people were certified to psychiatric units
there. That number includes people who were first arrested and then sent
from a detention center to a psychiatric unit. Approximately 20 percent
(1,380) of these patients went on to have civil commitment hearings. The
rest either signed themselves in voluntarily prior to the hearing or they
were released from the hospital before the commitment proceedings.
Of those who went to a civil commitment hearing, 1,165 (84 percent)
remained committed against their will, while the other 16 percent were
released by the administrative law judge who heard the case. Some were
released because of technical errors in the paperwork; others because the
judge did not believe they met the criteria for civil commitment. In 2012
the total population of Maryland was just under 6 million.

In California during the period from fiscal year 2000–2001 to fiscal
year 2005–2006, in the 28 counties that reported quarterly data, 593,751
people were admitted to the hospital involuntarily on what is called a
"5150," which refers to the section in the California Welfare and Institutions Code that provides for the 72-hour involuntary hold. The 28 counties
were inhabited by 22 million people, or 65 percent of the total population
of California. A little division and extrapolation yields an estimate of more
than 100,000 people who were placed on 72-hour holds during each of
those years in California alone. Thirty-four percent of those people were
then retained for 14-day holds, called "5250s."

Civil commitment procedures vary from state to state, although they
share some principles. In Maryland, patients can only be sent to a psychiatric unit involuntarily if they have a mental disorder and are judged
to be dangerous to themselves or others. The term "dangerous" is broadly
construed and can be interpreted to mean an inability to care for one's
basic needs, but most Emergency Department physicians interpret it to
mean that danger—or death—must be imminent. Two physicians or

psychologists must examine the patient and agree that he or she can't be managed in a less restrictive environment. An initial mental health evaluation occurs in the Emergency Department before a decision is made to admit patients, and they are given the option to sign in voluntarily if they have the capacity to make medical decisions.

In California, where Eleanor lives, the procedure is different. According to the Lanterman-Petris-Short Act of 1967, a single physician or a law enforcement official may hospitalize a patient for up to 72 hours, as Eleanor's ED doctor did. In California the law explicitly spells out that someone may be involuntarily hospitalized even if they are not imminently dangerous by using the grave disability clause. A mental health evaluation is not required before the admission, and Eleanor reported that the ED doctor spoke with her for only a few minutes. Because a psychiatric evaluation is not required before the patient is admitted to the hospital, it is not surprising that California has a high rate of involuntary admissions from Emergency Departments.

During those 72 hours, the patient has a psychiatric evaluation, and one of three things happens. The patient may be deemed safe enough to release, he or she may agree to sign in voluntarily, or a "certification for intensive treatment" (a 5250) can be instituted, at which time a hearing is initiated. If the patient is not released by the judge at the hearing, he or she can be held for up to 14 more days.

How often is someone certified to a psychiatric unit for an initial period of observation in other states? The frustrating answer, as already noted, is that we don't have good national statistics on this. Ted Lutterman is with the National Association of State Mental Health Program Directors Research Institute, and when I communicated with him in 2013, he confirmed that there are no statistics on the national rates of involuntary psychiatric hospitalization.

"After all the recent tragedies of violence by people with mental illness, we've gotten a lot [of] questions, and there is the assumption that state authorities must know the rates of involuntary hospitalizations," Lutterman said. "But when we've talked to states, we've found that many don't get that information."

Eleanor described the hearing she attended that allowed for her continued hospitalization: "I was in solitary that day, lying on the floor, thinking I was going to die. They came in and pulled me out and brought me to the judge. The doctor was there and a nurse. I wasn't asked anything. There was no lawyer. My husband wasn't there. I asked later why he wasn't there, and they said they had called the house and no one answered. I wasn't lucid. Then they had carte blanche to keep me for a long time. I was not offered representation."

With a court order granted, Eleanor was held for 14 more days.

Eleanor's psychiatrist, Dr. Green (not his real name), did not remember Eleanor. He had worked on the unit for nine years, and many patients had come and gone. He may well have been dismayed to hear that his patient was an example of those who feel injured by their care.

Dr. Green insisted that a hospital-appointed patient representative must have been present; he could not recall ever attending a hearing where one was not present. Eleanor's medical records contain no documentation of the hearings, so the story is one person's word against another's. There are signs on the unit, he noted, spelling out patients' rights, including the right to representation.

On September 13, Dr. Green applied for temporary conservatorship, also called "T-con," which would allow for another 30 days of hospitalization. The public defender's office appointed an attorney for Eleanor, and a second hearing was set for September 21. As it turned out, she was discharged on that date, and the hearing never happened. Eleanor says she was not informed of the application for temporary conservatorship and only became aware of it when she requested her medical records after her discharge. She felt violated because she did not have a way to advocate for herself. Furthermore, Eleanor thought her husband should have been included in the process.

Lily was hospitalized in Ohio, where patients are initially detained on a "pink slip," the state's lingo for an involuntary hold. She met with an attorney but did not attend her commitment hearing because she felt it was part of a plot against her. She was given paperwork indicating that the hearing had occurred and that she was committed to the hospital. Her brother, Joe, was not there either, and neither of them knows what transpired at the hearing.

In Ohio, before a commitment hearing is held, there is an investigation to consider alternatives to hospitalization in light of the allegations made in the affidavit. A report is submitted to the court, and a hearing is generally held within five days. Indigent patients are given counsel and even an independent psychiatric expert. Other interested parties are allowed to attend the hearing at the discretion of the judge. If committed by the judge, the patient can be held for up to 90 days without further review of the need for hospitalization. Unlike some states, Ohio law shows some sensitivity about how a person should be treated when taken to the hospital and specifically notes that the patient must be told that the detention is not a criminal arrest.

Lily said she was not handcuffed or treated harshly during the short drive from her home to the hospital. "There was no big confrontation. I was super psychotic."

If she had chosen to go to her commitment hearing, she may well have been transported by a sheriff to another site—either a courthouse or a state hospital—for the hearing.

In 2015 Dr. Joshua Sonkiss, a forensic psychiatrist and assembly representative to the American Psychiatric Association from Alaska, queried his colleagues and proposed an APA action paper to create a consensus on where civil commitment hearings are held. Sonkiss wrote:

> Courts in many jurisdictions hold civil commitment hearings at the hospitals where involuntary detainees are hospitalized. However, some courts transport patients from the hospital to the courthouse. Even where hospitals have facilities to conduct hearings on-site, patients are sometimes transported anyway as a matter of convenience for the court. Patients are transported in the same manner they would be if they had been arrested, charged with a crime, and transported to jail—a barbaric practice.
>
> Courts that transport patients for their own convenience may offer a list of excuses for not changing their policies to accommodate clinical considerations such as avoiding re-traumatization of civil detainees. One of these excuses is that there is no published consensus among psychiatrists as to the preferred location for civil commitment hearings. This Action Paper is intended to establish such a consensus. It is intended to protect patients' rights and ensure they suffer as little psychological harm as possible during the civil commitment process.

This action paper passed in the APA's assembly unanimously, but the consensus among psychiatrists does not mean that state laws will change.

It's easy to focus on the treatment of patients; many have stories about how they were egregiously wronged during their hospitalizations. One person, however, contacted us to say she'd been traumatized simply by the loss of her rights, despite being treated well when she was hospitalized after a suicide attempt:

> After reading other people's accounts of their hospitalizations, I can appreciate just how well treated I was at my hospital. The nurses and techs were kind and respectful, medications were not forced on me — they were strongly recommended, but I was allowed to refuse them. I was not strip-searched or restrained in any way, and the facility itself was comfortable and well funded. There was even a swimming pool. I couldn't go in because of my stitches, but I could sit on the side and dangle my legs in.
>
> And it was still one of the most traumatic experiences of my life. Even though I wasn't mistreated, I was still locked up against my will. It was terrifying to suddenly have no voice, to be transformed from normal college student into someone who was "mentally ill" and therefore unable to determine what was best for myself. I knew that I didn't belong in the hospital, but my thoughts and feelings meant nothing. It's hard to describe just how scary it is to be treated as if you are crazy, and know that there is nothing you can do to prove to the other person that you are not.
>
> After my 72-hour hold was up, I thought I would be released, but they told me they had filed papers to keep me indefinitely. I had been easy-going and pleasant up to that point. Even though I knew I didn't belong in the hospital, I could understand why they put me there, but hearing them say that was totally surreal and awful, and I stopped cooperating. I requested a lawyer, saw him the next day, and a few hours after our meeting I was released.
>
> Once I got out, I had nightmares for years about being back in the hospital. I tried not to think about what had happened, but the knowledge that my agency and voice could be taken from me at any time dominated my thoughts for years afterwards. I still managed to finish college, go to graduate school, and become successful in my career. I think the worst consequence of the hospitalization was that it scared me away from any

contact with mental health professionals for a long time afterwards. It is only in the last few years that I have started seeing a therapist again, and I feel sad that I went so many years of my life without help because of my experience at the hospital.

Do state laws that make it easier to forcibly admit patients make a difference in issues that might be meaningful to the average citizen? States vary with regard to their criteria for civil commitment. As mentioned, in Maryland an evaluation is done before admission, and two physicians or psychologists must certify that the patient is mentally ill, dangerous, and unable to be voluntarily admitted or treated in a less restrictive environment. In California, one physician can admit the person for 72 hours, and the evaluation is done afterward, on the inpatient unit. In some states, patients must be dangerous, while in others the criteria include being gravely disabled, meaning that because of a mental disorder, the person is unable to provide for his or her basic needs, including nourishment, shelter, and medical care. While the gravely disabled clause should make it easier to admit a patient to a psychiatric unit in California, the fact remains that every night in San Francisco alone, more than 4,000 people sleep on the streets while another 1,500 or more reside in shelters and safe havens. A large percentage of these unfortunate people suffer from serious psychiatric disorders.

People continue to die of hypothermia, and people continue to exhibit psychotic behavior in the streets. Apparently, making it easier to force treatment does not eliminate the phenomenon of people "rotting with their rights on," a phrase coined by forensic psychiatrist Thomas Gutheil in a 1979 article co-authored with Paul Appelbaum. Nor does it eliminate violence by people with mental illnesses.

Finally, we want to make the point that homeless, desperate people with mental illnesses often seek voluntary care and are discharged from Emergency Departments. While federal law requires EDs to evaluate patients, there is no standard for what constitutes being psychiatrically stable, and as we discuss in chapter 8, patients who seek admission to psychiatry units are often turned away.

Lily recognized that she was too sick to participate in decisions about her care. Eleanor asserted that her rights were violated, that she was not given reasonable representation, allowed to call witnesses, or given the opportunity to prepare testimony on her own behalf. Most laws regarding civil commitment are precise and thoughtful with a clear intent to protect the civil liberties of those involved. But sometimes, things go wrong. In the next chapter, we look at the history of civil commitment laws and talk about a case in Vermont where things seemed to spin out of control.

Christina Schumacher and the History of Civil Commitment Laws

6

"They all made the decision before I even arrived that they were going to check me in . . . check me into the mental health facility—a woman that just experienced the hell of her life," Christina Schumacher said in her testimony to the Vermont legislature in January 2014.

"That night, I went through the fires of hell just dealing with what I went through. And I may not be crying right now, because I have cried so many tears, in the psych ward, by myself, for fucking five and a half weeks, locked up. My family turned against me. I didn't even have the support of my own sisters and brothers; instead, they wanted me to be locked up and put on medicine."

The story, as reported by the *Burlington Free Press*, started with unthinkable tragedy, the kind of tragedy that makes some people put the newspaper down in disgust while compelling others to seek out more gruesome details. For this chapter, we use facts and quotes as they were reported by the media; we did not interview members of the Schumacher family.

Ludwig "Sonny" Schumacher was a former member of the Vermont Air National Guard. He had once been an air force colonel and an F-16 pilot. He had a law degree and a master's degree, and he had managed the reelection campaign for Vermont's lieutenant governor in 2004. Clearly, Sonny Schumacher was smart, talented, educated, and well connected.

His wife, Christina Schumacher, is, by anyone's measure, a beautiful woman with long hair and a perfect smile, and she worked for more than two decades at GE Healthcare. The couple, who looked like they danced off a wedding cake, were married for 19 years and had a son and a daughter. Their story should have ended with "happily ever after" but turned instead to cataclysm.

The Vermont couple separated, and in July 2013 Christina Schumacher obtained a "relief from abuse" order against her estranged husband. The order mandated that Sonny stay away from his wife and from their home and that he limit his contact to the email communications necessary to arrange for visits with their children. Apparently a judge did not find the children to be at risk, though the media would later report that Mrs. Schumacher repeatedly notified authorities that she had concerns about her husband's violent and erratic behavior.

According to news reports, on December 16, 2013, Sonny Schumacher made changes to his will, removing his wife as his heir and naming his sister as executor. He then sent documents to family members by FedEx, timing them to arrive on December 18. On December 17, he notified the school that their son would not be in attendance for two days.

We will never know exactly what happened after that, but the events as reported certainly imply that what happened was premeditated. On December 18, 2013, the bodies of both father and son were found in Sonny Schumacher's apartment, victims of a murder-suicide. Schumacher had strangled his 14-year-old child, then hanged himself.

"He strangled my son to death. Just that experience alone is more than any mother should have to bear. I'd never wish it upon anyone," Christina Schumacher testified before the state legislature, wearing dark sunglasses and a black cap over her long blonde hair. Even grief-stricken, she was a striking woman with a bold personality.

She continued with her testimony: "The next day, I had a lot of friends' support. I had a regular therapy appointment. I figured it would be a logical thing to do to actually go to that therapy appointment. So I made the choice to go."

Christina Schumacher said she was greeted at the appointment by her therapist, another psychiatrist, the clinic director, and two security guards. She was taken to Fletcher Allen Health Care, where she was hospitalized involuntarily on a psychiatric unit.

Nearly two weeks passed, and Mrs. Schumacher remained involuntarily hospitalized. From the hospital, she contacted the *Burlington Free Press* and asked the newspaper to investigate her case.

Another three weeks passed, and on January 24, 2014, after a three-hour hearing, Vermont Superior Court judge Kevin Griffin ruled, "The application for involuntary treatment is DENIED." Christina Schumacher was released from the facility, and days later she gave her testimony to the Vermont state legislature.

Schumacher was one of more than 30 people to testify before the legislature about proposed changes in the state's involuntary treatment laws. During the 2014 legislative session, a proposed amendment to Vermont's legislation required a shorter time before the civil commitment hearings that allow hospitals to hold patients against their will and also a shorter time before a separate judicial proceeding to allow facilities to involuntarily administer medications. The amendment was quite controversial. On the one hand, hospital beds were in short supply, and delaying involuntary medications kept people confined for longer periods. On the other hand, many saw efforts to speed the process as a move to clear beds faster, without giving patients a chance to come to their own decision with regard to continued hospitalization and medication.

It is generally agreed that it's better, and less traumatic, if patients participate in treatment of their own accord. No one was clear on exactly how much the amendment represented a reasonable attempt to facilitate patients' due process in a timely manner, and how much it was a financially motivated move to get patients in and out of the hospital faster. The two issues—the time before a civil commitment hearing and the time before a second hearing to permit the involuntary administration of medications outside of an emergency situation—were intermingled in the amendment, and Vermont is a state where both psychiatric and judicial resources are already overtaxed.

Schumacher testified about some of the problems she saw with her environment and with her care. "I fought for my rights and I'm out of there, and no one should ever have to go through what I've gone through. It has been hell, and I will not stop fighting this fight!"

The dire distress Christina Schumacher endured was obviously outside the scope of usual human experiences; we don't think of psychiatric units as places we involuntarily hold people who are grieving. Of course, there may be more to this story than was reported by the press. It's possible that the doctors and the patient's family had reason to believe that she was at risk. For the purposes of this chapter, however, we focus on the process of involuntary admission rather than the events leading up to it.

Specifically, we wonder how it could be that a patient was held for five and a half weeks without a hearing. As we saw with Eleanor, in many states psychiatrists may hold a person for a certain amount of time to assess the patient's need for continued hospitalization. That time frame varies among states but is usually days. This period allows for a number of things to happen, including careful observation and a full psychiatric evaluation. In many cases, there is an outcome other than a hearing. Patients may agree, for example, to a voluntary admission—either because fears of the psychiatric unit are dispelled once they have been admitted, or because the patients come to realize that they would benefit from the treatment being offered, or because they perceive that they would lose at a hearing. Other times, with observation, the psychiatrist does not feel the patient meets the criteria for involuntary commitment, and the patient is allowed to sign out of the hospital. If the doctor does decide continued hospitalization is necessary, there must be a civil commitment hearing, which takes some time to arrange, usually days, as mentioned above.

Dr. Margaret Bolton was the president of the Vermont Psychiatric Association in 2014. She is a forensic psychiatrist with an interest in commitment laws, and she spoke with me about the culture of hospitalization in Vermont. While almost every state has a shortage of public hospital beds, Vermont's difficulties were compounded when the Vermont State Hospital was flooded by a storm in 2011, and the state lost dozens of beds.

Bolton said, "We've had a robust advocacy group, and involuntary care is the last resort here. We have no separate forensic facility, and our state hospital washed away in Hurricane Irene. It's a real problem to find beds, and people get backed up in the ED, sometimes for *weeks*. We have a very high tolerance for risk and uncertainty, and we don't have a lot of bad stories. To get into the hospital here takes an act of God. We joke that it's easier to get into Harvard." There is irony about how difficult it is to get a patient into a facility for treatment (including treatment they want), and how much harder it may be to get them out. Bolton confirmed that once set in motion, the process of involuntary treatment and due process could be quite slow in Vermont.

"It is commonly 60 to 80 days to a commitment hearing," she said. "There is an amendment to the law to mandate a hearing within five days, and the judiciary is against it. There aren't enough judges. Now they are trying to mandate for a 'paper review' in five days and a hearing within 20 days. It almost doesn't matter what's written; what matters is how it's interpreted."

In Vermont, as in many other states, a facility has 72 hours to apply for involuntary treatment, which was formerly offered only in the Vermont State Hospital in Waterbury. The state facility housed more than 1,700 patients at its peak occupancy in the 1930s. During Hurricane Irene in August 2011, 51 patients were forced to the second floor by rising water and had to wait for rescue teams.

In situations like the Schumacher case, where the facts as given by one side seem to indicate an egregious betrayal of the patient's best interests, psychiatrists are often portrayed as having ulterior motives. Antipsychiatry groups contend that psychiatrists lack empathy or, worse, enjoy "power trips." Finally, some note that psychiatric facilities get paid for having patients fill their beds and may have a conflict of interest when it comes to releasing patients. One commenter on a patient bulletin board wrote, "Psychiatry is about money and power. When you bring it down to what it really is and what it's about, what it stands for and WHAT IT'S DONE; it's a money and power trip."

In light of the historical overuses and abuses of civil commitment, the right to a hearing remains a crucial part of the process. Dr. Daniel Fisher of the National Empowerment Center came at these issues from the vantage point of being both a psychiatrist and a former patient who had been hospitalized against his will. Fisher was the medical director of a community mental health center for 25 years and noted, "I did commit people at times when there was nothing else available. It's not a black-and-white world."

"The most astounding thing," Fisher said, "is that once you are labeled 'mentally ill,' you are no longer covered by the Constitution! There is no such thing as a 'commitment hearing.'" Fisher implied that such hearings may be done in a going-through-the-motions way in many instances.

"There is no opposing point of view and there is no independent psychiatrist at the hearing. Massachusetts prides itself on being liberal, but for a 20-year period, I was one of two psychiatrists who would even consider taking such a case."

Fisher said it was not unusual for the appointed attorney to meet the patient five minutes before the hearing. "I once said, 'You haven't even talked to the person.' The lawyer said he wasn't paid to do that. There is no due process."

Fisher felt that being held in a psychiatric hospital was sometimes related to finances:

> If you have the misfortune to have good insurance coverage, you often stay longer periods of time. And in military hospitals, there isn't even the pretense of a hearing; you're just ordered in and then ordered out. There's a board that meets. I was on the White House Commission on Mental Health, and we couldn't touch that. Unless you're on the other side of that locked door, then you just can't appreciate that there is no justice. Once you're deemed mentally ill, it's incumbent upon the person to prove they're not mentally ill, and that's almost impossible.

Christina Schumacher's case was finally heard. A Superior Court judge listened to three hours of testimony from both sides before he determined she should be released. One can only assume that it added to the patient's misery that her case was not heard in a more expeditious manner, which might have allowed for a quicker release.

As much as current laws have inconsistencies, looking back through history it's evident we've come a long way with respect to patients' rights. In early nineteenth-century America, before psychiatric hospitals existed, there was no consideration of patients' rights and no need for civil commitment procedures. People were cared for in their homes or left uncared for on the streets. Mentally ill people in jail were housed under filthy conditions, often chained to a wall or otherwise restrained.

When Pennsylvania Hospital was opened in 1751, it was the first public hospital in the United States; it was designed to care for the sick, the poor, and the mentally ill residents of Philadelphia. The hospital's founder, Benjamin Franklin, and later the medical director, Benjamin Rush, placed humane care as a cornerstone for the treatment of the psychiatric patients admitted there. The facility was designed to provide recovery through quiet contemplation in a peaceful country environment, and patients were allowed the freedom to socialize and converse without the use of the physical restraints common at that time.

Families sought admission for their ill loved ones, and no legal barriers stood in their way: all that was needed was a family member's signature.

That almost sounds ideal—no emergency rooms, no long waits, no incessant negotiations to get a bed for a very ill person who needs care—but anything that sounds too good to be true probably is. As the hospital expanded, admissions also grew, and soon overcrowding became an issue. More hospitals were built, in large part due to the untiring efforts in the mid-nineteenth century of Dorothea Dix, who lobbied the US Congress to set aside acres of land to create the country's public psychiatric hospital system.

Plentiful hospital beds allowed psychiatric admission to be a quick and simple process. Too simple, however.

One case in particular, that of Mrs. E. P. W. Packard, called public attention to the problem of a "no questions asked" admission process. Packard was admitted to the Jacksonville Insane Asylum in Illinois in 1860 at the request of her husband after several years of contentious marriage. In her autobiography, *The Prisoners' Hidden Life; or, Insane Asylums Unveiled*, Mrs. Packard wrote:

> Another fact I noticed, that he [the doctor] invariably kept these sane wives until they begged to be sent home. This led me to suspect that there was a secret understanding between the husband and the Doctor; and that the subjection of the wife was the cure the husband was seeking to effect under the specious plea of insanity; and when they began to express a wish to go home, the Doctor would encourage these tyrannical husbands that they were "improving." Time after time have I seen these defenceless women sent home only to be sent back again and again, for the sole purpose of making them the unresisting, willing slaves of their cruel husbands.

Packard spent three years at the asylum. Finally, she was released at a hearing after public attention was brought to her case. The Illinois legislature conducted an investigation into her allegation that she was confined in spite of being perfectly sane. Packard and eight other married women who were also committed to the hospital testified before the committee about the circumstances of their admissions and the hospital conditions. Packard's autobiography was published in 1868. In the introduction she wrote, "The legalized usurpation of human rights is the great evil underlying our social fabric. From this corrupt center spring the evils of our social system. This corruption has culminated in the insane asylums of the nineteenth century. Let the government but remove this cause of insanity, and the need of such institutions would be greatly lessened."

As a result of the testimony of Packard and the other women, the state of Illinois passed a law requiring a hearing before any involuntary admission, and Packard worked to see similar laws passed in other states.

Unfortunately, the requirement to have a hearing did little to prevent the possibility of a faulty, improper, or capricious admission.

In 1962, 60-year-old Catherine Lake was found wandering around Washington, DC. She was taken to an emergency room and eventually admitted to St. Elizabeths Hospital. She was committed to the hospital after two doctors testified that although she wasn't dangerous, she had trouble with her memory and didn't know the date or where she was. She was eventually located by her husband and sister, but a court refused to release her to their care because they weren't able to supervise her adequately. The US Court of Appeals for the District of Columbia later said that in this case the judge overseeing the commitment was obliged to consider the "least restrictive alternatives" to hospitalization before committing someone. The court didn't free Lake, however, or require a new commitment hearing, but it did require the trial judge to have a new hearing to explore options other than hospitalization.

In addition to requiring a judge to consider alternatives to hospitalization, several other protections were put in place in 1972 in response to the case of *Lessard v. Schmidt*. Alberta Lessard was picked up in front of her residence in Wisconsin by two police officers and taken to a hospital for an emergency psychiatric evaluation. She wasn't present at the hearing where a judge ordered her held for 10 days based on the testimony of the police officers. At the end of that time another hearing was held, again without her being present, and she was committed a second time after two physicians testified that she had schizophrenia. The patient was unaware that either of these hearings had taken place and was given no notice of them.

Lessard hired her own attorney, but in spite of this representation, she was committed for another 30 days. The judge did not explain this decision other than to say that she was "mentally ill." Her counsel, Milwaukee Legal Services, filed a class action suit on behalf of all adult committed patients in Wisconsin, alleging that the commitment law failed to provide enough protection of the patients' civil rights. A federal district court agreed. In addition to considering alternatives to hospitalization, the court found that patients had the right to be given notice of their hearing, to be given notice of their rights, and to be represented by counsel.

After listing all the deficiencies in the Wisconsin civil commitment law, the court cited former Supreme Court justice Louis Brandeis: "Experience should teach us to be most on our guard to protect liberty when the government's purposes are beneficent. . . . The greatest dangers to liberty lurk in insidious encroachment by men of zeal, well-meaning but without understanding."

It's not enough, however, to place due process protections at the beginning of an involuntary admission. Once admitted, patients have a right to get out. As odd as it sounds, that issue wasn't addressed until the 1970s—more than 100 years after Mrs. Packard fought for due process prior to admission.

In 1957 Kenneth Donaldson was admitted involuntarily to a hospital in Florida. Although he repeatedly stated that he was neither mentally ill nor dangerous, he was committed as suffering from schizophrenia. He remained in the hospital for the next 15 years. Throughout his hospitalization he petitioned the superintendent annually for release, eventually with the help of Dr. Morton Birnbaum, an internal medicine specialist who was also an attorney and a patients' rights activist. Birnbaum filed a civil rights suit against the superintendent on Donaldson's behalf. Testimony showed that the patient was not dangerous and that there was a less restrictive alternative to hospitalization because he had friends willing to take him in. But Donaldson's release was denied every year.

The case eventually went before the US Supreme Court, which in 1975 held that "a state cannot constitutionally confine in a mental hospital, without more, a non-dangerous individual who is capable of surviving safely in freedom by himself or with the help of willing and responsible family members or friends." Thus, the standard for release became one of safety or nondangerousness. While the Supreme Court never clarified what the phrase "without more" specifically meant, the ruling has often been understood to imply that committed patients have a right to treatment.

Birnbaum's daughter, Rebecca, a psychiatrist, later wrote about her father's work. She described the case in detail:

[Donaldson] contacted my father from the Florida State Hospital after chancing across the New York Times article describing the "Right to Treatment" legal argument. Mr. Donaldson sought release from the hospital because, he claimed, he was receiving inadequate treatment.

Dr. [J. B.] O'Connor, the acting clinical director of the hospital and Mr. Donaldson's attending physician from the time of his admission in January 1957 until the middle of 1959, claimed that Mr. Donaldson was receiving "milieu therapy," which consisted of keeping him in a large room with other patients, for most of his time in the hospital. Mr. Donaldson had been confined to a locked room with 60 beds. Mr. Donaldson argued that for 15 years, he received merely "custodial care" but not treatment for the supposed illnesses for which he was admitted. Mr. Donaldson was routinely denied activities that would have contributed to establishing a sense of independence and responsibility, including grounds privileges and occupational therapy. In the 18 months that O'Connor was in direct charge of his case, Mr. Donaldson spent no more than one hour talking to him. During his first 10 years at the hospital, progress reports on Mr. Donaldson's condition were irregularly entered in his patient record at intervals averaging one entry every two and a half months.

In the original complaint, Mr. Donaldson, guided by my father, attempted to bring a class action suit on behalf of all of the patients on his ward. In addition to damages to Mr. Donaldson and to the class, the complaint sought habeas corpus relief directing the release of Mr. Donaldson and of the entire class and sought broad declaratory and injunctive relief requiring the hospital to provide adequate psychiatric treatment. (A declaratory judgement is an order that decides a disputed legal issue, while an injunction is an order that requires a defendant to make certain changes or to stop doing something.)

My father would exclaim in disbelief in later years that for 14 years, on 18 separate occasions before every Florida and federal court having jurisdiction over granting the writ of habeas corpus and before more than 30 different state, federal, and U.S. Supreme Court judges, he was unable to obtain a fundamental writ of habeas corpus for Mr. Donaldson.

Both sides in subsequent trial testimony agreed that Mr. Donaldson presented no danger to himself or to others, that he had never committed any dangerous acts, and that he had never been suicidal. O'Connor claimed that Mr. Donaldson was never released because he was concerned that Mr. Donaldson would be unable to make a "successful adjustment outside of the institution."

After 12 claims before state and federal courts and after four claims before the U.S. Supreme Court, Mr. Donaldson was finally granted an unconditional release by the hospital in 1971, at the age of 62. After discharge from the hospital, Donaldson returned to his hometown in Syracuse, New York, and worked there as a night clerk in a hotel while he wrote a book about his experiences titled *Insanity Inside Out.*

Kenneth Donaldson drew the attention and help of a vigorous and prominent civil rights lawyer, who petitioned for his release annually. Other patients weren't so lucky.

Ann Fasulo was committed to a hospital in Connecticut in 1951. Marie Barbieri was committed to the same hospital in 1964. When they were first hospitalized, their commitments were not for a defined time. By the time they petitioned for release after the US Supreme Court decided the Donaldson case, they had been hospitalized for 26 and 13 years, respectively. The Connecticut Supreme Court agreed that psychiatric patients had a right to a regular review of their need for continued commitment. Justice Joseph Longo wrote, "The burden should not be placed on the civilly committed patient to justify his right to liberty. Freedom from involuntary confinement for those who have committed no crime is the natural state of individuals in this country."

Under federal civil rights law, every state now is required to have a system to protect and advocate for the rights of individuals with developmental disabilities or mental illnesses. This requirement is facilitated by the National Disability Rights Network, an organization with branches in every state.

Jack McCullough heads the Mental Health Law Project at Vermont Legal Aid. He noted:

> There are a lot of parts of the system that are there to look out for what's best for the client. Often their family members are looking at that, [as are] the community mental health system, the hospital, and ultimately the

judge decides. But there's only one person in the system who stands up for what the client wants and that's the Mental Health Law Project. For a lot of people it's really scary. They often disagree with the reasons for having been brought into the hospital, they often think they can make it on their own without hospitalization, and they are concerned that they don't have anyone standing up and speaking for them, and it's important for us to be there.

McCullough said that in 2013, 572 patients were involuntarily admitted to hospitals in Vermont. Some were released in the first few days. The state filed to proceed with commitment hearings for 445 patients, the majority of whom either signed in voluntarily or were discharged before a hearing could be held. Fewer than 100 patients went to a hearing.

While Christina Schumacher's hearing lasted for three hours, Mc-Cullough noted that most hearings take less than two hours. The hospital calls witnesses from the community, usually the mental health screener who saw the patient, a law enforcement official, a family member, or a staff member from the person's residential facility. The hospital psychiatrist also testifies. In all the cases that the Vermont Mental Health Law Project tries, the charts (often hundreds of pages long) are reviewed, and an independent psychiatrist is retained to provide another opinion. If that psychiatrist agrees that the patient needs to remain in the hospital, which is often the case, then the independent psychiatrist is not called to testify. This degree of preparation is, as Dr. Fisher pointed out, rare, and it contributes to the slower process in Vermont. This system is in sharp contrast to the proceedings Eleanor described in California, where she was pulled from a seclusion room and taken to a hearing without a consultation with an attorney and without her husband present.

"I want to win every case," McCullough said. "We do what there is to do, but we also recognize that there may not be a strong defense because of the evidence." He noted that most of the time, the judges rule to retain the patient in the hospital. "It's an event when we win one of these cases."

McCullough estimated that patients are released by judges in less than 10 percent of cases. He talked about one case in which the judge decided a patient was safe to leave, and on his way out of the courtroom, the patient threw a glass of water on the hospital's attorney. Not surprisingly, the patient was called back and retained after all.

In the legal cases discussed above, some patients were admitted because they were mentally ill, but as in the case of Mrs. Packard, some were committed for less justifiable reasons. The result of the 2014 legislative hearings in Vermont, after many hours of contentious testimony, was that the procedures were changed to allow for expedited commitment and medication hearings.

We will never know what words passed between Christina Schumacher and her psychiatrist that led him to believe she needed to be kept in a psychiatric unit against her will during such a terribly difficult period in her life. The tragic irony of the story remains: Christina Schumacher spent five and a half weeks on a locked unit getting unwanted psychiatric care, while her late husband—a deeply disturbed and dangerous man—did not.

Four

THE HOSPITAL

The hospital was a way station, a purgatory. . . . I was amazed that the fantasies of self-destruction all but disappeared within a few days after I checked in and this again is testimony to the pacifying effects that the hospital can create, its immediate value as a sanctuary where peace can return to the mind.

—William Styron, *Darkness Visible: A Memoir of Madness*

While I was preparing to write my student note for the *Yale Law Journal* on mechanical restraints, I consulted an eminent law professor who was also a psychiatrist and said surely he would agree that restraints must be degrading, painful, and frightening. He looked at me in a knowing way and said, "Elyn, you don't really understand. These people are psychotic. They're different from me and you. They wouldn't experience restraints as we would."

I didn't have the courage to tell him in that moment that no, we're not that different from him. We don't like to be strapped down to a bed and left to suffer for hours any more than he would.

—Elyn R. Saks, TED talk, June 29, 2012

Scott Davis on Law Enforcement and Crisis Intervention Teams

In this chapter we focus on how people get brought to care and how society can intervene to make access to care easier and less traumatizing. Over the course of the next few chapters, we discuss what happens in the hospital, the medical decision-making process, and the legal methods involved in different types of involuntary treatment.

Lily, you may recall, refused to go for help, and her psychiatrist sent the police to bring her to the ED. While she went calmly, this is not the case with all patients. In addition, Lily noted that she was not placed in handcuffs. In some places, shackling patients for transport is routine, and the entire process can be embarrassing, uncomfortable (even painful), and distressing.

Because the police are often responsible for transporting involuntary patients to the hospital in the course of a crisis, law enforcement is a logical place to begin the discussion of how forced psychiatric care transpires. I chose to follow a crisis intervention officer for two reasons: Officer Scott Davis was willing to have me accompany him, and specific mental health training might well be a small part of the solution to the broader societal problem of how we treat the ill among us.

"I tell my officers, you're social workers, whether you like it or not, because they're not calling their therapists or psychiatrists at three in the morning and getting a response," Officer Davis said. "They call us, and we have to handle that call. We don't have a choice."

The Montgomery County Police Department is located in a large building set back from the road and off the beaten path in Gaithersburg,

Maryland, a suburb of Washington, DC. Montgomery County is noted for its wealth and posh, its top-notch public schools, and its proximity to the nation's capital. Nearly 58 percent of the residents over the age of 25 have college degrees, and in 2009–2013 the median household income was more than $98,000, making it the tenth richest county in the United States. While Montgomery County certainly has problems with crime, it's no surprise that it's considered to be a safe and desirable place to live. It's also no surprise that its government has been willing to invest resources in training its police officers in how to interact with people who may be mentally ill in an effort to improve the safety both of the officers and of people whose needs are different from those of criminals.

The county's Department of Health and Human Services has a well-staffed Crisis Center with 42 employees, including 3 part-time psychiatrists, for a population hovering around one million; many Montgomery County residents are also able to afford private care without relying on government-run centers or resources. The Crisis Center provides telephone and walk-in services 365 days a year, 24 hours a day, and includes a mobile crisis team that makes house calls. Services are provided at no cost and, according to the department's website, are available in English, Spanish, French, and Vietnamese. In addition, the center has six crisis beds. This is a level of care that is unheard of in many parts of the country, where the nearest mental health clinic may be hours away. Even in Maryland, only 3 of 24 jurisdictions have walk-in crisis services.

Scott A. Davis is the coordinator of the department's crisis intervention team (CIT). He is a strapping man with close-cropped hair who makes a point of not wearing a patrolman's uniform. In khaki cargo pants, hiking shoes, and a long-sleeved, black, rugby-style shirt with "Crisis Intervention Team" embroidered on one side and the emblem of the Montgomery County Police Department embroidered on the other, he looks more like a high school football coach than a policeman.

Davis likes to be in constant motion, and he talks at a rapid-fire pace. He told his stories with all the evocative details that make for compelling drama, and he remembered not only the events of the moment he was describing, but also the backstory of each person from long before Davis had entered the picture. Since I'd been warned that police officers don't talk easily about their feelings, I quickly realized I'd stumbled upon a gem of an officer, and he was certainly an expert and an advocate in the field of mental health crisis intervention.

"I basically connect the dots between the mental health system and the police department. If there's a mental health problem, they reach out to me," Davis said.

Crisis intervention training (CIT) is a 40-hour course to instruct officers on how to recognize and respond to people with acute psychiatric issues. Mental health training is strongly encouraged by the National Alliance on Mental Illness (NAMI) because there is a belief that such training decreases police aggression against people with psychiatric illness. Studies have shown that CIT increases the likelihood that a behaviorally disturbed person will be diverted for evaluation and possible services rather than being placed under arrest.

There is also evidence that trained officers have a better capacity to verbally de-escalate or "talk down" disturbed people and that they feel more confident in their ability to work with people who may be suicidal or psychotic. While CIT doesn't guarantee that police won't use force, there is some evidence to suggest that CIT officers use verbal interventions more often than do officers without training.

Unfortunately, there haven't been enough outcome studies yet to see if CIT prevents assaults or deaths for either the police or the patient. In Montgomery County and many other places, officers are not required to attend CIT.

Montgomery County uses the Memphis model of crisis intervention, which started in 1988 as a joint venture among the Memphis police, the local branch of NAMI, and two universities, the University of Memphis and the University of Tennessee. The Memphis Police Department's website explains the mission of its program:

The Crisis Intervention Team (CIT) program is a community partnership working with mental health consumers and family members. Our goal is to set a standard of excellence for our officers with respect to treatment of individuals with mental illness. This is done by establishing individual responsibility for each event and overall accountability for the results. Officers will be provided with the best quality training available, they will be part of a specialized team which can respond to a crisis at any time and they will work with the community to resolve each situation in a manner that shows concern for the citizen's well being.

In 2008 there were more than 400 CIT programs operating in the United States. In 2011 there were more than 1,000 CIT programs worldwide. While many police departments have adopted the training, program implementation is hampered in rural areas where there may not be sufficient emergency room mental health services, enough practicing mental health professionals, or even any nearby inpatient psychiatric unit or hospital. This is particularly problematic since one study of patients' preferences showed that a person in crisis would prefer to have a joint response by a police officer and an accompanying mental health professional rather than a response by a police officer alone. In Maryland, there were only five jurisdictions with CIT programs in 2014. One estimate is that across the nation, 15 percent of police forces have crisis intervention training programs.

The police are often the starting point for involuntary psychiatric treatments. If any person, either with or without a psychiatric problem, is violent or threatening violence, the police may be called. Police officers who arrive at such a scene have a number of choices. They can assess the situation, help the individual to calm down, and then leave the scene. If a crime has been committed, they can arrest the individual and take him or her to jail. Finally, if police officers believe that a person has a mental illness and is dangerous, in Maryland they can fill out an emergency petition (EP) and take that person to an Emergency Department for psychiatric evaluation. The person in question does not have to have committed a crime to be subject to an EP, but the police officer, who may well have had no training in mental health issues, needs to believe that the person is both mentally ill and represents a danger to himself or others. Davis noted:

> For years, the standard was such that you couldn't rely on third-party information, so if an officer responded to a scene and the consumer wasn't presenting as dangerous, you couldn't do anything. The house could be trashed, but if Little Johnny was sitting on the table saying, "I'm good, sir, nothing wrong here," he wasn't presenting with signs of mental illness so you couldn't petition him. In 2005, that changed, and you could use cred-

ible third-party information from parents, caregivers, or teachers. Otherwise, officers would say, "I didn't see it." And there is still that perception out there to some degree.

Physicians and licensed mental health professionals can also issue EPs. In addition, anyone can go to a district court judge and present their concern that someone in their proximity (a family member or roommate, for example) is both mentally ill and dangerous, and the judge can issue the EP. In a situation where a physician, mental health professional, or judge files the EP, the police are then dispatched to bring the individual to the Emergency Department for an evaluation.

In many locales, that is enough to enable an involuntary hold, but every state has its own emergency evaluation procedures and requirements. In Maryland, the EP requires an emergency evaluation, but the EP alone does not trigger an inpatient admission. In the ED, the patient is examined, and if hospitalization is deemed necessary but the patient does not agree to voluntary admission, two physicians or psychologists must certify that the patient needs admission. This process is known informally as being admitted involuntarily on "certs." If the patient is later retained at a hearing, then he or she is officially "committed." Sometimes there is discord if a psychiatrist in the community has the police pick up a patient on an EP and then the physician in the ED does an evaluation and does not agree that the patient requires an involuntary admission. The ED doctor serves as the gatekeeper to the inpatient unit, and this can be frustrating for a psychiatrist in the community who feels strongly that a patient needs involuntary treatment in an inpatient setting.

In most of these scenarios, the police are involved either in making the decision to bring someone to an Emergency Department or in transporting them after the petition has been filed.

I asked Officer Davis if he gets anxious when he responds to a call.

"All the time. If I'm going out on a call, it's likely a mental health call, and there's always the propensity for danger. It's more than the cat-in-the-tree calls, so I think it's very dangerous. I'm not stupid. I never go into a situation by myself, I'm not that kind of guy. But I do feel a bit like Teflon when I go out on a call. I'm not thinking about getting hurt."

The dispatcher's procedure is to ask about drugs or weapons at the time of the initial call, and all people being brought into custody are patted down. Later, I watched as Davis called for a female officer to assist him at the Crisis Center so she could pat down a female patient who was to be transported to the Emergency Department.

The Montgomery County Police Department offers CIT instruction four times a year, and Davis runs that training. The 40-hour course is taught over four days, from 7 a.m. to 5 p.m. Of the department's 1,252 sworn officers, 600 have taken the CIT course. One hundred civilian employees have also participated.

The first day is all lecture. Next we do an auditory hallucination exercise where we have headphones and MP3 players, and the officers have to multitask while they're hearing these voices. Then we do half-day lectures and start site visits. We send officers to Adventist Behavioral Health, a free-standing psychiatric hospital which is two miles up the road, and then to the crisis unit and to the jail. It's important for me to let them know the resources that are available so they know when someone's in the hospital, okay, this is where they go. Half the group does that, and the other half goes up to Springfield to tour the state hospital. The next day, they actually have consumers come in to talk with them.

Davis talked about how he became interested in crisis intervention work. "I was good at doing it, not intentionally; it just kind of happened. You have to realize the consumers didn't sign up for this. They didn't say, hey, I'm gonna try the bipolar option. I don't have anybody who's mentally ill in my family, but I have a lot of empathy for these guys."

Davis may be an exception. One study that looked at the kind of officer who signs up for CIT found that volunteers were more likely to have had a personal experience with mental health issues and mental health professionals.

While there was no major mental illness in his family, Davis is no stranger to personal tragedy. His childhood was marred by the death of his 17-year-old brother when he was only 8. The brother was killed by a drunk driver, and the loss lingered over the family.

"After that, I was shielded. I wasn't allowed to do much; they kept me in the house a lot. Education wasn't really pushed. My dad was military police, and he would take me to work with him and I liked that. Then when I was 17 and a junior in high school, I went into a delayed enlistment program. I went to basic training after my junior year in high school and came back as a senior, did limited reserve training, and after graduation, I went to infantry training in Fort Benning, Georgia."

In addition, Davis started taking college courses while he tried to decide what he wanted to do. Before going to the police academy, Davis was a correctional officer at a jail for three years. He then was a police officer on a military base for another three years.

"We enforced both military and civilian laws. It was a lot of domestic violence, DWIs, a lot of shoplifting. Actually pretty boring work. And then a friend I met at DOD—Department of Defense police—left to work for Amtrak police in DC, and he recruited me. It was a lot of fun. Union Station was the most secure train station you'd ever find in the world when we were there. Everybody got locked up for everything: zero tolerance. We were a little crazy." Davis smiled as he talked about that time in his life.

Davis entered the Montgomery County Police Academy and spent 6 months in training, followed by 12 weeks of field training. He graduated from the academy in January 2003.

"This is a calling; you gotta want to do it. There are people who get 15 or 20 years into it and decide this isn't what they want to do, but they stay because they are vested and have benefits."

Davis's crisis intervention team was started in 2001 by Chief Charles Moose, who had come to Montgomery County from Portland, Oregon, where CIT had been introduced in 1995. The first CIT director was Joan Logan. She had a master's in psychology and had retired from the military as a major. Davis noted that she had excellent leadership skills. Logan was sent to Memphis for training.

"She came back, and she said this is going to save lives, and she said it's going to save *our* lives. When you talk police jargon, you always talk about our safety first. When we talk to the public, we talk about how it saves consumer lives, but that's just a little bit of word salad." Davis smiled as he spoke.

Logan ran the program until she was injured in a biking accident and then retired in 2010. Before she retired, she called Davis and asked him to take over as director.

"I had a really good history of doing [emergency] petitions. Especially coming from DC where in Union Station people with mental illness would come out of the woodwork. Knowledge of the process is first and foremost, followed by understanding mental illness."

Davis noted that in Montgomery County, CIT is required before an officer can be issued a Taser, or stun gun. Each stun gun costs the department $850–$1,000, depending on the model. While expensive, the Tasers are useful, Davis contended. "They've saved a lot of lives. They save consumers' lives. When they present a physical threat, it's very quick and humane, and there's no long-lasting effects. Once it's over, it's over. The officers will do the CIT training just to get the Taser, [but] then they'll tell me they got something out of it."

While Davis claims that Tasers are safe, their use has become a topic of controversy, and they have been associated with deaths, especially in people with preexisting cardiac conditions, which may be unknown to both the officer and the individual. There is a movement to limit their use to those situations where a police officer might otherwise use a gun and the results would clearly be lethal.

Being shot with a Taser hurts, and Davis reported that CIT requires that the master instructors—of which Davis is one—experience being hit with a Taser.

"They shoot you in the back with the darts, so the darts go into your skin, and you go down for the full five seconds. It knocks you on your ass, and it hurts. It's great for credibility in the courtroom. You can say, 'I do know what it does because I've been hit by it.'"

Montgomery County assistant police chief Betsy Davis (no relation to Scott Davis) commented on the changes she's seen with CIT, including a reduced use of deadly force and decreased officer injuries, which she attributes to the Tasers.

"More people in crisis are brought in to be treated, or at least to get an evaluation, as we are better trained and are seeking treatment for them, rather than entering them into the criminal justice system. We are spending more time with people in crisis as we have better training, but that puts the officers out of service for longer." In other words, the cost of diversion from the criminal justice system is in human resources. This is a theme we discuss in later chapters about the inpatient unit and about efforts to minimize the use of physical restraints.

When a call goes out that there is a person with possible mental illness, there is no protocol in Montgomery County to ensure that CIT officers are dispatched to the scene. For the most part, it's a matter of chance as to whether people with psychiatric problems end up having CIT officers respond to them. That being said, while he was driving, Davis continually checked his computer screen to see what calls were coming in so that we could go to the scenes of any that were related to mental illness.

When I do education in the community with NAMI or with consumer families, I tell them if it's a mental illness–related call, they should request a CIT officer. You'll hear it on the dispatch — complainant wants a CIT officer — and that puts the officer on notice that the person requesting police services knows that CIT officers exist and that there's probably an expectation of better service. That's my strategy to put the program out there and to validate it more. That way, if there's a lazy cop — it's a small percentage, but we have them — then if he's thinking "that's a crazy coot, tell them to make more hats with aluminum foil" so he can clear the call — I'll tell them instead to request a CIT officer.

Davis said that in 2013 the Montgomery County PD responded to 5,256 calls related to mental health and substance abuse issues. That was up from approximately 4,250 calls in 2012. The officers, he noted, were given wide latitude to decide what to do about nonviolent offenses committed by people with known or suspected mental illness. This pre-booking diversion attempted to funnel people away from jail and into treatment, and it involved a lot of behind-the-scenes relationships with NAMI and the mental health community. In fact our day had begun at 7:30 a.m. at a meeting of the Montgomery County Criminal Justice Coordinating Commission, where Davis was one of the speakers.

Davis drove an unmarked gray sedan, and, as already mentioned, he intentionally did not wear a uniform. "I wear this because I get a lot further when I do interventions. People don't want to talk to you when you wear that uniform. My shirt still says 'police' and still has a badge, and I still have handcuffs and all."

He gave me a tour of his trunk and his jump-out vest. In addition to his service Glock, a Taser, and an M16 assault rifle, Davis traveled with a flashlight, handcuffs, a trauma kit, and rifle plates for his bullet-proof vest. There was also a device to deflate tires for cars blocking the road. "Standard stuff, everyone carries this," he explained.

The communications were constant. He had a smartphone and a lap-top mounted in the car. A dispatch radio made intermittent announce-ments. When he wasn't communicating with someone else or talking with me, he watched the streets and ran license plates on the laptop while he was stopped at intersections. Overall, he maintained a level of vigilance and activity that I found exhausting. All things considered, it was shocking what a good driver he was, and when I commented on this, he replied that he was being more careful for my benefit. I let him know I appreciated that.

One of the major complaints about involuntary hospitalization is that the process can be upsetting and humiliating. People are handcuffed and escorted to a patrol car, sometimes in front of their neighbors, co-work-ers, or family members. At the Crisis Center, Davis and another police officer handcuffed a patient to bring her to the Emergency Department. They made a point of telling her repeatedly that this was protocol and that she had not done anything wrong. It helped that while she was dis-organized, manic, and agitated, she was cooperative and did not resist any of their maneuvers; my sense was that this was not the first time the police had transported her to an emergency room.

The two officers helped the woman into Davis's car, displacing me into the back seat for the short ride, and told her how to hold her hands to prevent discomfort. At moments during the brief ride, she was agitated, upset, and loud. At other times, she was calmer and talked about her sister, who also had a mental illness. Davis uncuffed the woman as soon as she was settled at the hospital.

"The unpredictability of mental illness dictates that we have to do this to be safe. There's no other restraint yet; handcuffs are it."

Mental health dispatches, he noted, are always called as emergencies, even if the original contact is from the Crisis Center for a patient who is calm and cooperative.

"If a patient tells the therapist he's thinking about killing himself, they'll call the police for a transport, and that goes out as a lights-and-siren re-sponse. I'm trying to get the dispatch supervisors to change that, to make it not an emergency response. If someone has a knife to their throat, then that needs an emergency response."

Davis shared some of the frustrations with his job. He didn't like being the lowest in the pecking order in the chief's office. His ideas, he noted, were sometimes dismissed.

"What I do is very nontraditional. It's very hands-on, it's very action-oriented, it's very time-intensive, and some officers don't get it. They think, 'I'm here to be a cop, to write tickets, to stop a bank robbery.' We get those calls too, but it's a very small percentage of what we do. Most of the time, we're interacting with emotionally disturbed clients in the field. I've dealt with them right on that sidewalk. Here," he said, pointing to the pavement where I was standing with him in a strip mall. "They are everywhere. This irritates a lot of people. The fact is that I specialize in a certain skill. It's a skill that's becoming very chic and very sexy nationwide, and everyone wants a CIT now. And as long as I'm the coordinator for the program, it's not good enough. It has to keep getting better."

Davis discussed the public's perception of police work during interventions with people with mental illness.

People just start berating the police. One woman was talking about one day she wasn't doing anything wrong and police officers just threw her on the ground, handcuffed her, and took her against her will to the hospital. She said the police response was just horrible; they didn't know what they were doing. She wasn't sick, and everything was fine. And I thought, wait a minute, you're here and you're alive today because of what the police officer did. There's two sides to every story, and if you lack insight and you're uncooperative, you would be thrown on the ground. No one throws someone on the ground who's cooperating. We take people down, but we try to go as easy as possible. Even with the kid gloves I use, people sometime go down hard. A lot of these individuals—because there's a mind-body disconnect with the dopamine in the brain—they'll fight right through whatever we're doing, so you have to use a lot of force. You have to put them down hard. That's just the nature of the beast. No one likes doing it. She talked about that nonstop, but there would be so much more credibility if she came to the table with a solution.

Davis talked about bringing patients to the hospital for evaluation. There are hospitals he likes and hospitals he doesn't like. Some of them, he felt, treated him with more respect and considered his input, and they got the patients seen faster. Other times, he was frustrated. He'd bring in a dangerous patient, and the hospital wouldn't restrict them, and the patient would escape. He'd then be called back to hunt down the same dangerous patient.

Davis said it was important to document why a patient needed to be in the hospital. When we had dropped off the patient at the Emergency Department earlier, he told the nurse that she had threatened suicide to the crisis counselor. He made a point of leaving his card along with the paperwork and told me he'd return for the commitment hearing if his testimony was requested.

I asked how a police officer decides to bring someone either to the hospital for a psychiatric evaluation or to jail to be charged with a crime. Davis told me that for nonviolent offenses, it was the police officer's discretion. For minor, nonviolent crimes, such as urinating in public or disorderly conduct, an officer might take a patient to the Crisis Center rather than either arresting him or taking him to the Emergency Department. "Trespassing is the biggest thing; we deal with that more than anything."

Law enforcement involvement is often the point at which the decision is made to initiate the process of civil commitment. The police officer, who may have no training whatsoever in mental health issues, or 40 hours of training in a best-case scenario, may be the one deciding whether to leave a scene or to take a person for a psychiatric evaluation. Outcomes get measured in many ways, but perhaps the most important result is the one that's hardest to measure. It's here, at this entry point, that a patient begins the difficult journey of involuntary care. If the process is respectful and gentle, the patient may get help without anger, humiliation, fear, or traumatization. If the event is violent or humiliating, the door opens to what may ultimately prove to be a distressing episode and one more reason to fear mental health interactions.

The physical danger is real, both to the citizen and to the police officer. Davis has never fired his service revolver or injured a patient, and his sensitivity to mental health issues is remarkable, but that result is not simply from 40 hours of training. He has supplemented his crisis intervention education with evening college courses in addictions and psychology, and his language and skills reflect much more knowledge than anyone could glean from a four-day course.

While police shootings involving mentally ill people are widely publicized in the media, national statistics have not historically been kept on how many people are killed by the police. Police officers also have been injured, or even killed, in their dealings with people who suffer from mental illnesses or are intoxicated. According to the FBI's Uniform Crime Reports, in 2012, 48 law enforcement officers died from injuries incurred in the line of duty when responding to reports of felony crimes. Only one officer was killed while handling a person with mental illness. Eighteen of the assailants were under the influence of drugs or alcohol at the time of the murders. Of all the arrest-related deaths reported to the Bureau of Justice Statistics between 2003 and 2009, 89 (1.8 percent) of the detainees' deaths took place during a mental health transport.

Compton and colleagues reviewed the literature on CIT in 2008. There were only 12 methodologic studies, and most involved the effect of training on officers' knowledge and skills related to mental illness. The CIT officers were more likely to feel well prepared to deal with calls involving the mentally ill and to view the mental health system as being helpful. A later Compton study showed substantial improvement in the officers' de-escalation skills and improved decision-making regarding referrals to mental health services. While crisis intervention training didn't predict the level of force that would be used in an encounter, it did increase the likelihood that the individual would be referred for mental health services or transported to a mental health facility rather than arrested. It also increased the likelihood of voluntary transport to a mental health facility. The studies emphasized the importance of having close coordination between the law enforcement and mental health systems, and the need to have community services readily available. While CIT programs reduced the money spent on criminal prosecution and incarceration, the amount spent on mental health services increased—making the programs cost-neutral.

To find out how CIT works in another state, we looked at Miami-Dade County, Florida, which is home to the largest percentage of people with serious mental illnesses of any urban area in the United States. Over 9 percent of the population (more than 235,000 individuals) experiences devastating mental illnesses, yet less than 15 percent of these individuals receive care in the public mental health system. Law enforcement officers have become, by default, the untrained responders to people in crisis. On any given day, the Miami-Dade County jail houses approximately

1,200 individuals with severe psychiatric disorders at a cost to taxpayers of more than $65 million annually.

The Eleventh Judicial Circuit's Criminal Mental Health Project was established to divert nonviolent, psychiatrically ill defendants away from the criminal justice system and into community-based treatment and support services. Steve Leifman, the associate administrative judge for the Criminal Division, has been intimately involved with this transition. Judge Leifman is fond of telling audiences, "When I became a judge, I had no idea I was actually becoming the gatekeeper to the largest psychiatric facility in the state of Florida. And while it sounds funny, it's sad, because it's the Miami-Dade County jail."

Leifman talked with me in 2014 about his experience with CIT in Miami-Dade County. They have had a CIT program for almost 14 years. "When we started this, there was great reluctance among law enforcement to do this. They didn't think they needed it, and they didn't like civilians telling them what they should be doing. It was quite a battle at the beginning. I remember going to meet with the police director and telling him they needed to do this. He returned and told me they'd checked their system and they only get about *five* mental health calls a year, because of course they didn't track them as mental health calls at the time."

With time, tracking, and more accurate classification, Leifman concluded that an accurate count of calls related to mental illness and substance abuse was closer to 5,000 per year for this particular agency. There are 36 separate police agencies within Miami-Dade, including the county police. Countywide, law enforcement in Miami-Dade handles approximately 19,000 CIT calls per year. Leifman was able to get Miami to slowly start the program.

"The city of Miami had a horrible situation where the police shot a Vietnam vet. They shot him 13 or 14 times, and this was after I was asking for this program. He had severe PTSD and mental health issues. They then kicked into gear, and they started to do a really great program."

Following this incident, a grand jury was empaneled to study the problem of people with mental illnesses caught up in the criminal justice system.

"It was a phenomenal report," Leifman noted. He provided testimony to the grand jury, which included some recommendations. The report described police shootings and the deaths of people with mental illnesses, and concluded that these were inappropriate.

"We started a massive training of everybody in Dade County after the grand jury report came out, and it has turned out to be one of the most successful endeavors I've ever been involved with."

In Miami, there are now more than 4,100 police officers—30–40 percent of the force—trained in crisis intervention. There are trained officers in all 36 agencies, in the county, and in corrections. There is a CIT coordinator who has developed an executive training program—which they use in addition to the Memphis model, "to teach the brass at each agency how to run CIT. The internal workings of an agency [don't] necessarily know how to run it, to juggle schedules, to make sure all neighborhoods are covered 24/7, every day of the week, with no gaps. In addition, there are 911 call-taker trainings to teach them how to identify mental health calls and dispatch a CIT officer right away."

What impact has the growth of CIT had in Miami-Dade, an area that's admittedly rougher around the edges than Montgomery County? The two largest agencies, the City of Miami Police Department and the Miami-Dade Police Department, keep data on every CIT call they make. Combined, the two agencies handle approximately 10,000 CIT calls a year.

"Last year [2013], the City of Miami Police Department handled about 5,000 calls, and out of those 5,000 calls, they only made 5 arrests, used very little force, and had no police injuries. This is amazing. There were 1,200 referrals to crisis units."

Leifman and I talked about whether changing how the police react to disturbed people has the potential to make police-initiated care less traumatic.

"There's a huge, palpable difference. In most of the cases, the police who've been trained know how to talk, they know how to avoid an involuntary hospitalization by just using verbal skills. They de-escalate, they keep it calm so the person doesn't necessarily need an involuntary, or they get the person to voluntarily take treatment. It's significantly better."

Leifman said that the CIT program has had an enormous impact on the jail census. The jail census, rather than a prison census, is used to assess outcomes because a jail houses criminal defendants who are awaiting trial or who are serving only short sentences. A prison is a facility where people serve long sentences after they have been convicted or pled guilty to crimes. People with serious mental illness who commit minor crimes are much more likely to be in jail than in prison, so the effects of a CIT program will be seen first there. The number of people in the Dade jail went down from 7,800 to fewer than 5,000, and a jail was closed last year [in 2013]. In addition, the city of Miami went from 12–14 shootings of people with mental illness annually before CIT, down to only a couple over the past few years.

Leifman doesn't believe that all police officers should be trained in CIT. "As one of the captains once said to me, 'Not everybody is meant to be a SWAT officer and not everyone is meant to be a CIT officer.' If you [are] trained but you're not sensitive to it, it doesn't work. We have a four-hour program for everyone to [learn how to] keep things calm until a CIT officer gets there, and that works for us. They go out of their way not to make threats, not to use force. We have very few shootings, and we used to be among the worst."

Leifman mentioned that the coordinator gets roughly 250 calls a month from the CIT officers for their own mental health issues. "You talk about trauma, and what we didn't appreciate beforehand is that these officers have their own trauma. I will tell you it's helped them immeasurably, and they feel great about the program and better about themselves. It's been an amazing cultural shift in my community. Every year, there's a ceremony to present an award to the CIT Officer of the Year. Approximately 500 people attend. They get up there and they cry giving speeches."

Leifman went on to say that he is not against involuntary treatment. In Florida, the initial step to an involuntary hold is called the Baker Act. "The key is not waiting for people to get so sick that we have to involuntarily hospitalize them. The key is maintaining people in treatment so they don't need involuntary hospitalization."

Leifman does not know if diverting people from jail to the mental health system has changed the rate of involuntary hospitalization. He cited hassles and headaches for the doctors, who must go downtown for the hearings, and he noted that 150,000 people annually are "Baker Acted" in Florida, of whom only 1 percent go on to a commitment hearing. The criterion in Florida is "imminent dangerousness," and the "self-neglect" clause is never used.

"In Florida, we have no money," Leifman said, noting that the state's per capita spending on mental health care is forty-ninth in the country. "If someone is sent to a crisis unit more than twice in a year, there's an

85 to 90 percent chance they'll end up getting arrested. There's a direct correlation between not getting people services and criminalization."

Leifman said there was some interesting positive fallout from the CIT program: the mayor of Miami went to New York to get the city's bond rating improved.

> After a three-hour presentation on the growth of the economy, they only had one question for him: they wanted to know how we got our police shootings down so significantly. And why would that be important to bond raters? Because the municipalities and local governments were self-insured, [and] whenever they would shoot and kill someone, there was a lawsuit that invariably followed. The city was paying hundreds of millions of dollars in lawsuits that came out of the taxpayers' bottom line, and with CIT we stopped it, and it improved the bond rating.

CIT programs are met with positive regard, and NAMI campaigns to have these programs incorporated into local police forces, but I had to wonder what the programs cost. When I asked both Judge Steve Leifman in Miami and Assistant Chief Betsy Davis in Montgomery County, the answer was surprising. Both said the costs were negligible. There is the salary for the CIT coordinator, the cost for the officers who conduct the training, and the labor replacement for the 40 hours that an officer is in class.

Officer Scott Davis was clear that he sought more liberal laws to allow involuntary treatment of the mentally ill, and he favored forced care. He saw forced care as a good thing, not a traumatizing one. He may not have realized how far his gentleness might go in preventing a sense of violation when he explained to a patient that he had to cuff them, that it was routine procedure, and that they hadn't done anything wrong. Unfortunately, as he noted quite vividly, it doesn't always go smoothly.

Does CIT teach police officers to behave in ways that are less traumatizing to patients even when care is forced? We just don't know because so far no CIT outcome studies have asked the patients about their attitudes and experiences.

Montgomery County, Maryland, is an exceptional place with exceptional people and exceptional services. It is not a microcosm of life in America, nor are the services offered for mental health or the training programs for law enforcement officers indicative of care in the country as a whole. Davis provided a glimpse into his world, a world of education, resources, and notable sensitivity. Meanwhile, Judge Leifman in Miami provided balance by talking about a completely different experience—an urban setting with a high proportion of people with serious mental illnesses where mental health services are severely underfunded.

In both settings, crisis intervention teams have made a positive impact. To us, 40 hours of training for the frontline responders for our nation's sickest—and sometimes most dangerous—individuals seems pitiful. What's even more shocking is that there is still hesitation and resistance to adding this small effort to the mental health care system when the paybacks can be so high.

Leonard Skivorski and the Emergency Department

Eleanor's experience in the Emergency Department was frustrating. She sat for eight hours.

"They put me in a cubicle in a plastic chair, all alone, and they came in and out and asked me questions. They kept grilling me about my medicines. I hadn't eaten or slept, there was no food, and my husband was told to wait outside. They didn't do anything. I don't know what that was about. Finally, we just left."

On the ride home with her husband, Eleanor was exhausted and emotional. "I went into a nonstop monologue and confronted Frank about everything that was wrong with our 20-plus-year marriage."

Frank offered to take Eleanor to another Emergency Department. She agreed it was a good idea, so instead of going home, they went to another hospital. In the parking lot, Frank asked Eleanor if she was feeling suicidal.

"I cracked," Eleanor said. "I went from being in control to being psychotic. Screaming came out of me from some depth, and I grabbed on to him. I was shrieking, as though another person were there. I almost didn't have a 'myself.' There was overwhelming fear, and I had gone over the edge. In the ED, they took me immediately with no waiting. The terror was so unlike anything I had ever experienced. I was afraid I would kill myself. I was irrational."

Frank said he felt compelled to ask his wife if she was feeling suicidal because he'd been in psychiatric treatment twice in the past, and he had entertained suicidal thoughts. His second psychiatrist had diagnosed him with bipolar disorder and treated him with lithium, which Frank had stopped taking soon after he and Eleanor were married. That psychiatrist had asked for reassurance that Frank would not commit suicide, reassurance that Frank had given. Confused by Eleanor's distressed state of mind, Frank asked her about suicide because of his own past thoughts.

"I had to ask," he said. "If I took her home and she harmed herself, I would never forgive myself." Frank's experiences in treatment were both positive. He had found psychiatry to be helpful, and he trusted his doctors.

In the Emergency Department, Eleanor was given an injection of Ativan, a sedative that is similar to Valium. She described the doctor who gave her the injection as gentle and kind. Almost immediately after the injection, she felt much better. By this point, however, a decision had been made to admit Eleanor to the hospital. Lab tests were done, Eleanor had an MRI of her brain, and then she was transferred by ambulance to a nearby private psychiatric hospital.

The Emergency Department is the portal to nearly all inpatient commitments. It's there that the decision to admit or discharge is made, and the staff then pivot an unwilling patient in one of two directions: to the inpatient unit for involuntary hospitalization or to the exit door. The decision to release or admit a patient may literally be one of life or death.

The ED is a place where emotions are intense. Patients can be very sick, distressed, and demanding. Many of them leave unsatisfied. While the patient may have one agenda, the family may have another, and even when there is a clear solution, the resources are often unavailable.

The events in the ED can be ugly to observe. In emergency psychiatry, the first goal is to stabilize agitated patients enough to talk with them. This may require getting a patient into a physical space that is safe for both the patient and the staff, and may entail the use of physical restraints or placement in a seclusion room. Stabilization may include injecting patients with medications to calm them down. Some patients are violent; they may be responding to hallucinations. Other patients are intoxicated. For patients who are calm and able to converse, the question is often reduced to whether it is safe to let them go, or whether they should be admitted to a psychiatric or substance abuse facility—if one exists and if space is available. Most patients are released with a referral for outpatient treatment. With the exception of administering medications to calm an agitated patient, little goes on in a psych ED that would be deemed "treatment." The ED is a place to contain someone and make a decision about the need for admission.

With all these issues in mind, I asked the psychiatry resident I spoke with to remain anonymous. He was willing to use his real name and the name of the institution where he is in training, but I worried that this might compromise his ability to speak openly, and I wondered if there could be consequences for his career. He chose the pseudonym Dr. Leonard Skivorski.

Skivorski exuded a degree of self-confidence that is common in young doctors. He spoke with the bravado that doctors use when telling each other their war stories but later worried that he should have been more cautious with what he said. He is bright and energetic, and he obviously cares deeply both about having his colleagues know that he is working hard and doing a good job and about doing right by his patients.

In a teaching hospital with a psychiatry training program, the psychiatry emergency area is generally staffed by residents like Skivorski—young doctors who have completed medical school and are now learning to be psychiatrists. The resident reports to an attending physician, a doctor who has completed all of his or her training and is more senior. In the ED, the attending is usually an emergency medicine physician—someone who is specifically trained to work in this intensive setting and deal with all types of medical and surgical emergencies—and not a psychiatrist.

The psychiatry resident gathers the history, does the full assessment of the patient, orders medications, and decides whether the patient requires admission or not. Ultimately, if the resident decides a patient needs to be in the hospital and the patient refuses admission, the resident is the person who admits a dangerous patient against his or her will. In effect, the most crucial decision in psychiatry is often entrusted to the professional with the least experience.

Skivorski walked me through life in the psych ED. He began by describing the structure of the department in a hospital with a psychiatry training program. In this setting, there are resources available. The hospital has both a psychiatric unit and outpatient programs to which patients can be referred. In many, if not most, community hospital EDs in the United States, however, there is no access to a psychiatrist, and decisions about a patient's disposition are left to the emergency medicine physician, who may consult with a case manager or social worker rather than a psychiatrist with medical training, as we discuss in more detail later in this chapter.

Skivorski described an unspoken understanding between the emergency medicine attending physician and the psychiatry residents about what constitutes a reason to seek a consultation in an emergency setting.

> That understanding gets complicated. On one hand, the ED doc should be able to care for simple psych problems without consulting us. For instance, if someone is not in danger but has a probable anxiety disorder, the ED doc should be able to reassure them that they are right in seeking help and give a referral to an outpatient clinic. Or if a patient comes in for a medical reason but also has schizophrenia and is out of meds, they should be able to recommend that the patient restart his medicines if they were already prescribed. But when it's suspected that someone is suicidal, or if a patient is floridly psychotic, they should consult with psychiatry. Often they call us for anyone with any whiff of a psychiatric problem, including personality issues or problems getting along with their care team. If someone says they're having a panic attack, the patient is supposed to get medically cleared and get an EKG and labs. Then, often what happens is the ED attending calls us and says he thinks it's a panic attack and asks if we'd like to eyeball the patient. Usually what we say is, "No, it's an inappropriate consultation." They should provide resources for an outpatient psychiatrist, if the patient is interested. We're not going to do a full evaluation on this person in the ED for panic attacks at 4 a.m.

While that may sound a bit callous, Skivorski was referring to the fact that a panic attack is diagnosed only when testing reveals that the symptoms are not caused by something else, such as a heart attack. The end result—referral for ongoing outpatient care—will be the same whether or not the patient has an evaluation by a psychiatrist in the ED.

"Once I had a really bad consult," Skivorski continued. "We weren't busy. It was pretty quiet, and after I got up to the call room to get some sleep, they called for a consult for 'sex addiction.' The guy had come in for hypertensive crisis [severe high blood pressure], but it turned out to be caused by crystal meth. He mentioned he had a sex addiction, and the emergency medicine doctor wanted a psychiatry consult. This just isn't something that's going to get treated in an emergency room."

A young woman, Elizabeth (not her real name), told me her experience in an Emergency Department in another state. Her husband had called the police to bring her to the hospital the day after she'd threatened suicide. She had just learned she was pregnant with twins, and in her state of heightened emotions, she had not meant her threat to be taken literally. She was shocked when her husband involved their parents, his own psychiatrist, and then the police. She was taken to an ED, evaluated, and ultimately released. Although no one had abused her, Elizabeth remained distressed about the event many months later. She had been seen by both a social worker and a psychiatry resident in the ED.

"I realized I had to think about how I answered every question, and I couldn't allow myself to get angry," Elizabeth said as she tended to a crying infant, one of the twins who had since been born. "They talked to my husband and to my mother without me, and I knew they were going to make this decision as though I were a child. But I had gone to work that day, and I was a functional adult. I realized I was stripped of any agency. They were condescending, and there was no kindness."

Elizabeth is still experiencing distress, and even though she was not involuntarily hospitalized, she remains uncertain about the future of her marriage.

Dr. Kevin Klauer is the chief medical officer for Emergency Medicine Physicians, a group that staffs 70 Emergency Departments across the country. He estimates that he has worked in 10 different EDs over the last 15 years in Ohio and Pennsylvania. Klauer said that in most of the settings where he's worked, there is no access to a psychiatrist, and there are not residents in training, like Dr. Skivorski, to help with the assessment and disposition of patients in a mental health crisis. He calls for a mental health consultation only after he has determined that a patient needs hospitalization, and the consultant is often a case manager without medical training whose job is to facilitate the patient's admission.

Klauer elaborated on some of the points Skivorski made.

If someone comes in with an anxiety disorder and they aren't suicidal, I'm not going to call a mental health worker. But if someone has a life-threatening mental health presentation, then they need to have that level of consultation, and we're going to ask for it every time. If someone is suicidal, I can't think of a time I would send them home. I'm very cautious about letting someone go home when they've changed their mind about being suicidal. I let the mental health professional make that decision, but when it comes down to it, if I am the physician of record, then I have to be accountable. So I give great deference to a mental health professional, but I don't give them the complete latitude to discharge our patients. I'll say, "Because of what I've heard, I'm not comfortable discharging them." Once that flag is raised and I'm worried about someone, why wouldn't we err on the side of giving them more services and not less?

Klauer's point is a good one, and it comes from his motivation to keep patients safe and to do his best to care for them. It does not, however, take into account that a patient could leave feeling injured by the intervention, as Eleanor did, or have the lingering distress that Elizabeth has.

"I'm never going to trust a mental health professional again; I just could never do that. I'm learning about how the mental health system functions and what the laws are so that I can protect myself from ever going through this again," Elizabeth said. She told me she knew she was at risk for postpartum depression, having just had premature twins, and she didn't know what she would do if she became depressed down the line.

Skivorski listed the three ways patients come to be seen by the psychiatry resident in the ED. "First, when they come to the ED, if they say the word 'suicide' to the triage nurse, or if they seem completely psychotic. Second, if they are admitted to the medical side and a psych complaint comes up. And finally, if they come in with the police specifically for a psychiatric evaluation."

Common reasons for emergency evaluations include suicide threats or attempts, public nudity, accosting people on the street, or decompensation into psychosis or mania. In these instances, the patient may be responding to hallucinations or delusions and behaving in a bizarre manner. Skivorski estimated that between one-third and one-half of the patients in the psych ED arrived with the police.

"Some of the patients brought in by the police are there voluntarily— they've asked someone to call the cops on them to get the ride!" A police escort is free while an ambulance may come with a bill.

Elizabeth said that when the police arrived at her home, she did not realize that she could refuse to go to the hospital and they legally would not have been able to take her. Her family would have had to get a court warrant. Instead, the police called an ambulance, and she was brought in as a voluntary patient, even though she didn't know that.

"We get emergency petitions for weird reasons," Skivorski said.

> This past Saturday, I saw a guy who had no psych history. He was soliciting men for sex, and the cop who picked him up brought him to the ED. He said, "This guy is going to get beat up if he goes to prison so I'm bringing him to the hospital instead." If we see them and we clear them for discharge, we don't call the cops back to take them to jail. So it ends up being much less paperwork for the police, but it also saves someone from having to go to jail. I don't know the legality of it. The cop took pity on the guy, but this patient was really pissed off that he'd been dragged into the hospital. I don't think he realized the other option was jail.

Given that the ED can be an unpleasant and stressful place, it would be easy to imagine that all patients are there against their will. In *Mad Science: Psychiatric Coercion, Diagnosis, and Drugs*, authors Stuart A. Kirk, Tomi Gomory, and David Cohen discuss coercion and voluntary psychiatric hospitalization:

> We conservatively estimated that around 1.37 million adults are the subjects of involuntary hospitalization each year. This number makes up about 62 percent of those hospitalized for any psychiatric reason but does not include the unknown proportion of those deemed to be "voluntarily" hospitalized but who are aware that they might or will be forced into hospitalization if they do not submit. Our own guess is that the large majority of psychiatric hospitalizations, perhaps all, are involuntary.

While every psychiatrist would agree that some patients who sign into the hospital voluntarily do so because they have been persuaded, coerced, or even threatened with involuntary commitment, there are still many people who come to the ED actively seeking voluntary admission.

In the course of researching this book, we found that people often didn't know if they had been admitted against their will. They may have been told they had to go to the hospital—in much the same way that someone having a heart attack or in a diabetic crisis is told they have to go to the hospital—and then signed themselves in. Technically, this isn't involuntary care; it's following a doctor's orders and being a good patient, even if there are other places that person might rather be.

Some patients related that they truly did not want to stay, but were told that there was no choice and that they could physically be held against their will and committed by a judge unless they "chose" to sign in. While this is clearly coerced care, for this book we hold to the standard that a judge needs to order the treatment for it to be truly involuntary. Thus, the perspective expressed by Kirk, Gomory, and Cohen in *Mad Science*—that *all* patients admitted to the hospital are there by force—is unnecessarily inflammatory and simply inaccurate. The issue, however, does get quite murky.

People seek voluntary admission through the ED for a number of reasons. It is where people go when they are seriously ill, often with profound depression or acute psychosis, and have nowhere else to turn. Access to voluntary care is an enormous problem in the United States, and even those who are insured may have trouble getting to see an outpatient psychiatrist. It's not unusual to wait three to six weeks or longer for an appointment with a psychiatrist—an unthinkable length of time for someone who is suicidal or suffering from paranoid delusions.

A 2014 study published in *Psychiatric Services* showed that even in major cities—Boston, Houston, and Chicago—where it is typically much easier to find care, it can still be difficult. Researchers posing as patients—either with health insurance or willing to pay out-of-pocket for treatment—called for an appointment with a psychiatrist using the Blue Cross provider panel as a reference. They were only able to get an appointment 26 percent of the time. Access to treatment is even more difficult in rural areas and for patients with no health insurance. In half of all counties in the United States, there are no mental health professionals (not just psychiatrists) at all. Access to voluntary care is terribly difficult.

Unable to find timely care, patients may come to the ED in search of voluntary treatment. The sad irony is that people who want to be admitted are frequently turned away because there are not enough beds or because insurers have set the bar for admission so high. Those who aren't actively dangerous often can't be admitted even if they come begging for help.

This lack of outpatient resources was highlighted by Ira Burnim, the attorney for the Bazelon Center: "By the time people are so deeply in crisis, there aren't a lot of practical options left, and they end up in the hospital."

Another reason patients may want to be hospitalized from the ED is to evade an unpleasant living situation. Skivorski talked about one woman who sought admission to a psychiatric unit because she was concerned there might be bed bugs in the group home where she lived.

Finally, there are those who seek voluntary admission because they are in need of drug or alcohol detoxification, or because they are homeless and have nowhere safe to sleep. This group of patients is sometimes referred to—in an admittedly dismissive fashion—as wanting "three hots and a cot." These people often know that if they threaten to commit suicide, they will be admitted. Their relationship with the ED staff may become adversarial, and the staff may well try to make the patient uncomfortable so a suicidal statement will be retracted. Skivorski said:

> The major issue is with substance abusers. We have "frequent flyers" who use EDs regularly. I try not to admit people who are just saying they're suicidal to get a bed. It's a bad thing to do because it encourages that behavior and then those beds can't go to patients who need them. For every patient we admit, a really sick patient is going to be left waiting in the ED for many hours, and someone isn't going to get care. But the reason we sometimes do admit them is because the medical attending will say, "Listen, this guy is saying he's suicidal. Even if I believe he's not dangerous, if he leaves here and gets hit by a car, it's in the record that he was suicidal."

Skivorski confirmed what Klauer had noted: psychiatrists are more comfortable discharging patients who say they are suicidal than emergency physicians are.

It's ironic that, on the one hand, forced care is held up as a way to prevent homelessness, violence, and incarceration, and on the other hand, society does not want to voluntarily hospitalize and treat homeless people.

Skivorski went on to discuss situations in which patients are brought in by a family member, but they don't want to be admitted.

> We have people who want us to certify their schizophrenic family members, but the patient is stable and has outpatient care. The family may not be happy with their level of care no matter what services are in place. They

may say that the patient is still sick, and she should be in a hospital. We'll hear, "We went to the trouble of getting a judge to authorize the evaluation so we want you to certify her." But she is at her baseline, and she wants to leave, so I let her leave. If the patient and the family are in agreement, usually we do what they request. I don't think I've ever certified someone whose family didn't want them admitted. If someone needed to be in the hospital and their family was against it . . . well, I've never been in that situation so I don't know what I would do.

From a psychiatry resident's perspective, a bigger issue is how to deflect people who seek admission for reasons other than an appropriate use of inpatient beds. Given the high rates of death from unintentional drug overdoses and the high rates of violence associated with substance abuse, it's remarkable that society draws a distinction for involuntary care: it can be used for mental illness but not for substance abuse issues alone in most states. Addiction, perhaps, is assumed to include an aspect of choice.

There are always concerns about liability if a patient is released and there is a bad outcome. Dr. Klauer, who also has a law degree, talked about the possibility of being sued for malpractice.

I haven't heard of a lot of medical-legal cases where someone was let go and then killed themselves. What I have found is that if you have really performed a good-faith evaluation, and despite that, there is someone who truly wants to harm themselves, eventually they are going to find a way to leave the hospital, and they are going to harm themselves. They may tell people what they want to hear to let them go. It's a very sad statement for a very small subset of patients. However, if someone was evaluated well, and everyone was in agreement with letting them go, there isn't much more you can do.

While there are many components that factor into a psychiatry resident's decision to hospitalize a patient—voluntarily or not—another aspect is the pressure to release patients. There are people who are in distress who want inpatient treatment but do not meet the medical necessity criteria set by insurers for inpatient treatment. Insurance companies may require that a patient be acutely dangerous or may insist that a cheaper level of care would suffice. Psychiatry is the only field of medicine where someone's life must be at risk for a hospitalization to be authorized by the insurance company.

One woman I spoke to in California was hospitalized involuntarily after a suicide attempt. I asked why she didn't sign herself in, since it seemed obvious that a judge would keep her after an overdose had landed her in the intensive care unit. "The doctor said my insurance would only pay if I went in on a 5150," she responded.

In a similar vein, both Skivorski and Klauer told me that if they have to transfer someone to another hospital, they send the patient with forms for an involuntary admission, even if the person is willing to be admitted voluntarily. The concern is that if the patient changes his or her mind during the ambulance ride for the transfer, then a dangerous voluntary patient must be allowed to leave.

Finally, peer pressure plays a role in the decision a resident makes to release a patient. "You don't get [negative] feedback if you release someone you shouldn't have," Skivorski said. "We get in more trouble for 'soft' admissions: we get feedback from our peers if we admit someone who didn't need to be admitted. If you send someone out who belongs in the hospital, it's likely that no one's going to know—we never hear about the majority of bad outcomes. So residents go home at the end of the day either thinking they did a great job or worrying about every little thing."

Despite the uncertainty of it all, Skivorski said he doesn't lose sleep over these issues. "I'm an arrogant guy, so I err on the side of thinking I probably made the right decision. If I'm on the fence about someone, then I tend to admit them."

Semantic differences, or differences in how the law is interpreted, can also determine who gets admitted involuntarily and who gets released. Skivorski explained the training he received regarding the legal criteria for involuntary admission. In his state, the law allows for involuntary commitment if someone is dangerous, but the statute doesn't define what exactly it means to be "dangerous," and clinicians interpret this differently.

We had a couple of lectures by a forensic psychiatrist. But also, we start[ed] in the ED as third-year residents, and the real training we received came in the second year, which [was] all done on the inpatient unit. We went to a lot of court hearings with our patients who were involuntarily admitted

from the ED, and we would hear a judge say why a certification was appropriate or inappropriate. From that, we developed a sense of who the judge
will keep in the hospital and who they will release. We were taught to use
a pretty broad criteri[on] for dangerousness, and that's what I've seen hold
up in the courts. A common thing in the inner city is that it's a hostile environment, so if you have someone who is going up to gang members and
accosting them, he is going to get himself shot, so we count that. Much
more often, it's about being dangerous to themselves. I can think of very
few people that I've certified for being dangerous to others. I'd say at least
90 percent of the time it's about dangerousness to themselves.

This was a figure that was consistently cited by psychiatrists when I
asked what percentage of patients they hospitalized for being dangerous
to themselves versus dangerous to others. They all said "at least 90–95
percent," and every psychiatrist I spoke with said it was uncommon to
see a patient who was dangerous to others.

While Skivorski said that he'd been taught to admit patients involuntarily with a wide latitude for defining dangerousness, I wondered if he
had ever stretched the definition to include someone he believed needed
treatment, but who did not meet the legal criteria. He responded with a
story about an elderly homeless man who was brought to the ED by the
police.

"When he was first brought in, he was swinging his fists, and we called
in the security guards. He kept saying, 'Let me outta here, let me outta
here, let me outta here.' We ended up having to B-52 him."

Skivorski explained that "B-52" is jargon for a sedating cocktail of
medications that is given to acutely agitated people in the ED: Benadryl;
Haldol, 5 mg; and Ativan, 2 mg. The purpose of giving this combination
is to quickly calm a patient down.

So he was lying in a seclusion room, and I went in and he said, "You bas-
tards better let me out of here!" He was screaming and ranting, and he
was disorganized and unable to be calmed. So I said, "Listen, I want you to
have a conversation with me, so I'm going to leave and come back when
we can have a conversation." And he said, "No, we can have it now because
I want to get out of here. If you're treating me like a prisoner, then you're
a Nazi, and then I'm going to talk to you like you're an animal." He said it

very calmly; it was a weird disorganization, and I was thinking this old man had a dementia. I called his son. I found him by Googling his last name. The son said, "Thank God! We've been trying to find Dad for a long time." The last time his kids had heard about him was months before when they were called after the father had been let go from another ED. "You have to keep him," the son begged.

The man had been ill for a number of years. His behavior had become strange and disorganized, and he'd been unable to pay his bills. He had lost his home, and none of the housing options that were presented to him were acceptable; it wasn't clear how he was surviving. His children would look for him, bring him back to their homes, and he'd leave.

"So we have this guy, and he wasn't a danger to himself," Skivorski said.

He'd proven that: for the last however-many months he'[d] been living in the same neighborhood. He was bruised up and he'd been getting into fights, but he wasn't on drugs, and he'd been eating somehow. So it was a hard call to say that if I let him go he wouldn't just go on surviving—maybe not thriving—but surviving as a homeless man. But his kid was begging, and I couldn't let him go. There's no hospital for that; no hospital wants demented patients. And hospitals are good at finding reasons not to take patients. I talked to his son, and I went through all the options of places that would take geriatric involuntary patients. I arranged for his admission, and I signed out to the resident coming on after me. I told him, "If there's a problem, call me and I'll wake up. I want him to stay."

It turned out they couldn't get the bed after all, so they decertified him and let him go. Since then, I see this guy almost every week at the farmers' market, sleeping on one of the benches, and he doesn't recognize me at all. I feel badly on both counts. I feel badly that I certified him because he did not meet the criteria, and that's been proven because he's still alive. But I also feel badly that he didn't get to go into the hospital, because I know the unit I was sending him to, and they would have set this guy up. They would have calmed him down—probably by using medicines that wouldn't have had bad side effects—and they would have placed him in an assisted living facility or on a locked geriatric unit. People do stay in locked units for the rest of their lives, and they would have found a place for this guy. I worry about him every time I see him.

Nothing about the emergency setting is easy, certain, or safe, but hearing these stories, I did think of Dr. Fisher's comment that he'd never seen a patient become violent without provocation. I wonder how much of what we've come to accept as normal and necessary in the course of emergency care should be reexamined with the intent of minimizing procedures that might provoke a distraught person.

We want to emphasize that the laws in different states can result in very different outcomes. In *Crazy: A Father's Search through America's Mental Health Madness*, journalist Pete Earley wrote about rushing his son Michael to the Emergency Department at Inova Fairfax Hospital in Virginia. During the ride, Michael was disorganized and incoherent. Although he initially refused to take his antipsychotic medication, he eventually swallowed a pill at his father's urging.

"God. Capitalism. Satan. Comic books. Sex. Spontaneous laughter," Earley wrote, describing the conversation in the car on the long drive from New York, where Michael was a student, to Virginia, where his father lived. And then Michael asked him, "Dad, how would you feel if someone you loved killed himself?" Earley had every reason to believe his son was dangerous.

In the ED, the Earleys sat for four hours before they saw a doctor. Eventually, the emergency room doctor explained that the Virginia commitment law required that the patient must say he planned to harm himself or someone else. But Michael denied to the doctor that he planned to hurt anyone, so he was released.

Dr. Thomas Wise is the chair of the Department of Psychiatry at Inova Health System. Wise confirmed what the doctor had told Earley. "The law at that time required that the person swearing out the detention had to hear from the individual that they were going to kill themselves or others. You could not use hearsay."

Sometimes, only tragedy can force stringent laws to change. In 2008, following a mass shooting at Virginia Tech that left 32 people dead and 17 wounded, the Virginia law pertaining to mental health care was changed. The new law altered the wording from a requirement for "imminent danger" to allowing for court-ordered treatment if there is the "substantial likelihood" that individuals would cause harm to themselves or others, or be unable to protect themselves from harm or attend to their basic human needs. The more important modification is that the law now allows a judge to consider "all relevant hearsay" evidence when making a decision about civil commitment. The doctor no longer has to be a firsthand witness to the dangerous behavior or threatening statement.

A reasonable person might also wonder why Earley's son had to wait four hours to be seen, and why he wasn't seen immediately by a psychiatrist. After all, no one would expect a seriously ill patient with chest pain to wait that long.

Wise said, "In Virginia, a physician or a psychiatrist in the ED cannot petition for involuntary admission the way a physician in another state can. Detentions and petitions for involuntary hospitalizations have to be done by a mobile crisis team that is located in a community mental health center."

So even if the doctor in the ED had determined that Michael needed admission, he would still have had to call a mobile crisis team to come to the ED to assess his patient and facilitate the admission. No wonder Pete Earley titled his book "Crazy."

Klauer added some perspective on what it's like to get psychiatric services for a patient in a hospital where there is no inpatient psychiatry unit.

"Every single evaluation is a struggle. It's a struggle because of a lack of resources and a lack of ability to get people plugged in. It's amazing to me [but] when you're in a community setting where there is no mental health unit, you have [to] work with what you have. Usually, a case manager comes from a local mental health department, and it can take them hours to come to do an assessment."

In many places this wait can extend to days, and in some places it can even extend to weeks, as in Vermont. The process of holding patients in the ED is called "boarding," and it can be extremely uncomfortable—*miserable* might be a better word—for patients to remain for extended periods of time on a gurney or in a seclusion room in the ED while a bed is located and treatment is delayed.

Klauer talked about boarding as a tragedy. He's seen patients wait for hours for a case manager to come to do the evaluation—12 hours, he noted, was not unusual—and then much longer for a bed to be available. It's a topic that gets him quite animated.

"Do they need a bed, or do they need treatment?" Klauer asked.

The point I'm trying to make is that if they can't be admitted, then why isn't there something we can do to help them? All too often, while mental health patients are boarding in the Emergency Department, they are not being treated for the illness. This is equivalent to a patient boarding with pneumonia [but] not receiving any treatment, such as intravenous antibiotics. [And] those patients that we are holding awaiting a mental health evaluation, the overwhelming majority are not admitted; they are discharged anyway. People can be boarded for days. It's horrible! It's embarrassing to all of us who practice medicine. If we can't accommodate them, then can't we get the right provider in front of them?

I can guarantee you that if someone came in with an ST segment elevation myocardial infarction [evidence of a heart attack], no one would care about the insurance, nobody would wait for a bed to be available. They would go right to the cath lab and get their PCI [percutaneous coronary intervention] and get the rest of it sorted out later. But if someone comes in with a mental health emergency and they are no longer at risk to harm themselves, because they are now in our care, we frequently don't have the resources to get them an evaluation or a bed in a timely manner. They sit, and they get no treatment. What other clinical entity do we treat that way? Nothing! It is really, really bizarre, and it's so upsetting to me that this is how we treat our mental health patients.

Klauer suggested that telepsychiatry, where a psychiatrist meets with a patient using video technology, such as Skype, might help address the shortage of psychiatrists in rural EDs.

In 2014, the Washington State Supreme Court declared psychiatric boarding to be unconstitutional in that state, though it was not clear where the patients would go. The Virginia law used to require that a bed be located for an involuntary patient within six hours or the patient had to be released, regardless of how ill or dangerous that patient might be. This particular Virginia law received national attention in 2013 when the son of state senator Creigh Deeds was released because no bed could be located within the six-hour time frame. Deeds's son returned home, slashed his father's face with a knife, and then fatally shot himself.

Wise explained, "One of the problems with Creigh Deeds's situation is that the mobile crisis unit had to come from a couple of hours away to a relatively rural hospital in the southwest part of the state to make a determination of dangerousness."

Wise noted that following the Deeds's tragedy, the regulations were changed to require state hospitals to take patients when another bed cannot be located, thereby eliminating the potential for this situation to occur again.

Hospitalizing a patient across legal jurisdictions can create an additional complication. Monica Taylor-Desir is a psychiatrist at the Salt River Pima-Maricopa Indian Community. In a workshop Dr. Taylor-Desir gave at the American Psychiatric Association's 2015 annual meeting, she noted that there is no hospital on the reservation, where she serves as one of two psychiatrists. If a patient is detained involuntarily on a civil hold, he or she is kept in the local jail until the evaluation is done and a bed becomes available at a nearby state hospital, which is outside the tribal jurisdiction. It's a process that can take weeks, and although the jail employs nurses during weekdays, on evenings and weekends care is given by correctional officers with no medical training. This is an unforgivable way to care for ill patients!

Earley's account of what happened in the Inova Fairfax Emergency Department illustrates what is wrong with a system that relies on forced treatment. In Earley's recollection, the ED doctor didn't even *try* to engage his son before declaring that there was nothing he could do. While the law may have prevented the doctor from committing Michael Earley, there was nothing in the law that prevented the doctor from at least attempting to coax the distressed patient into a voluntary admission. Based on a statement by the triage nurse that Michael believed that medications were poison, this doctor's job ended before it even began. Perhaps Michael could have been cajoled into signing himself into the hospital. He was, after all, already in the Emergency Department voluntarily at the request of his father. It's also possible that an interested doctor who spent some time with Michael might have come to appreciate the danger of his disorganized delusional state and decided that he could, in fact, be committed.

Can we imagine the response if a doctor told a patient he had cancer or needed life-saving emergency surgery, and the patient said he didn't want treatment? Wouldn't the doctor make an effort to explain why the treatment was needed and what the consequences might be of not having it? Wouldn't he enlist the efforts of the family to persuade the patient to comply with the recommended course of action? Of course he would. A concerned doctor wouldn't accept a perfunctory "No, thanks" and walk away, but Michael's ED doctor seemed to have entered the room with a predetermined mind-set: if he couldn't force the patient to have treatment, why bother?

Dr. Skivorski was comfortable with the standard he was using to certify patients to the hospital and with the outcomes he was seeing. I wondered if he was a little too comfortable, if ordering B-52s and restraints and being pretty sure most of the time about whom to force into the hospital came a little too easily. And I say that not to criticize Skivorski specifically, because having once been a young and inexperienced psychiatry resident in the ED with a half dozen or more very sick patients under my care, I know that when the morning came, I often counted my own survival as one of the victories. The ED is not an easy place to be.

To work in an emergency room, you have to have faith that what you're doing is right. There's a lot of work to be done—difficult work—and new doctors rely on their teachers and on senior doctors to tell them how to proceed. Leonard Skivorski is sure of what he is doing, because he's bright, excited by his work, and absolutely dedicated, and he has faith that there is a right answer. Kevin Klauer is equally certain that it's right to hold people who may be dangerous.

It wasn't until we started hearing from patients that we even began to question whether involuntary treatment might be problematic. As we've noted several times, there is no research: we don't know if committing people to the hospital prevents suicide and homicide or drives people away from getting care in the future, perhaps leaving them even more vulnerable.

In the case of someone who is acutely psychotic and disorganized, there is a place for involuntary commitment from the emergency room. When all else has failed, it is hard to imagine that letting people continue in their psychic torment is safe, reasonable, or humane. And it's especially hard to imagine letting someone walk away if we believe their discharge will result in an imminent death. We're left with the question of how to preserve the civil rights of one person to remain outside of an institution, while also providing for the right of another person—someone such as Lily—to get much-needed treatment in a kind and respectful manner.

Eleanor was admitted to the hospital, and she contends that her treatment was deficient. In reviewing her medical chart, I saw that during her weeks there her blood was drawn once to measure calcium, magnesium, thyroid function, and syphilis serology. A test for syphilis is routinely done on all psychiatric patients without regard to their sexual history because neurosyphilis can mimic a psychiatric disorder. I could find no evidence that a drug screen, routine tests to check blood count, or a chemistry panel were done, though it is likely they were performed in the Emergency Department before she was transferred. While the psychiatric medications she was given are known to cause hyperglycemia (diabetes) and to raise lipid levels, testing was not done to monitor those conditions during her hospital stay, and the only nod to lab work was a note in the admission orders that read "Do labs if not done in ED." If the ED labs were ever located, they were not included in the extensive medical records that Eleanor provided to me.

Is it relevant whether all the usual tests and procedures were done and checked? Several years had passed since Eleanor's hospitalization, and she ultimately did well. There were no awful consequences from not performing the lab tests, but because of their absence I gave Eleanor's story of being mistreated more weight than I might have if the hospital staff had been meticulous about following the usual protocols.

Eleanor was distraught at the time she entered the hospital; she wasn't sleeping, and soon after admission she began to have paranoid delusions that filled her with terror. To be more specific, she believed that a night nurse had been hired by one of her relatives on the other side of the country to kill her. The nursing notes document that she was disorganized, uncooperative, and talked nearly nonstop, "yelling, non-directable, intrusive with peers and staff." She was repeatedly placed in a seclusion room where she was "unable to follow directions, yelling, banging on window, banging on door, unable/unwilling to contract for safety." Nursing notes from September 3 justified the use of seclusion: "Aggressive with staff, trying to get the door; Assaultive to staff, unable to follow directions." At times, she jumped on the mattress and tried to cover the camera in the seclusion room. Two notes referred to Eleanor's assertion that she had "superpowers."

Eleanor was placed in seclusion numerous times through September 11. For several days after that, she continued to receive injections of medications for "extreme agitation." Eleanor felt mentally impaired by the medications, but her activity level remained elevated, and even with high doses of sedating drugs, she still required a sleeping pill to get rest at night.

Eleanor discussed how she perceived what happened. The day after admission, she was involuntarily injected with a sedative without an explanation of what she was being given. After that, she was terrified and refused to cooperate with the staff.

> Multiple orderlies would throw me down and give me shots. I genuinely thought the staff were trying to kill me when they grabbed me and injected me. I had no idea at all what they were injecting, and it absolutely terrified me each time. I lived through the injection, and I was amazed that I had survived, and yet I kept waiting to die during the first hour or so after. It is why I fought so hard to stay awake and continue to function, so I would live through the "lethal dose" they had injected. Sometimes they injected me in the calf, and it was very painful. One nurse said to me, "I'm purposely hurting you so you'll cooperate next time."

The nurse's statement was not documented in the chart, and there is no way to independently verify if it was actually said, but such vindictiveness by a nurse would be deplorable. Could such behavior truly exist among mental health professionals?

In her book *Weekends at Bellevue*, psychiatrist Julie Holland openly described her own heartless reactions to some patients. She watched a group of prisoners who were brought to the Bellevue ED for treatment:

> The prisoners, dressed in orange jumpsuits, their hands and legs shackled, will make their way through these back hallways towards the rear exit, where a bus is idling. It is the most abject, sorrowful group of men you will ever see.... When I first started at Bellevue, I was callous, posturing with bravado while I watched them pass. Sometimes I'd even whistle "I Love a Parade" as they went by.

Holland also wrote about how she threatened a patient with a specific medication: "He knows his drugs. He knows Thorazine will make him feel absolutely horrid. He knows I mean business, and if he's a good little boy, maybe he'll get a treat. I may feel charitable and give him one of the sedatives on his wish list. But if he's bad, he'll get the charcoal in his stocking."

Such treatment of ill people is sickening, but it does exist, and health professionals in all fields, not just psychiatry, do sometimes rationalize mistreating patients.

The orders on Eleanor's chart allowed that the medications could be given by injection if she refused to take them by mouth. Eleanor says there were times when she was injected without first being offered medication in pill form and that she was injected even when she was not behaving in a threatening manner. Eleanor's interpretation of the events includes the possibility that it might be a normal response to become distressed, suspicious, fearful, and angry after being repeatedly and violently restrained by four men, then injected with unknown medications that sedated her. She has a point.

Eleanor described her experience of psychosis in vivid terms: "It was a dream state, even though you're awake, but the interpretation is distorted by the dream state. Whatever is happening, there is an explanation that the mind fills in to make it real, [but] the explanation might not be right. Then it will morph and become a completely different scenario, and what I was thinking about would be a transitory, ever-shifting episode. But like a dream, it [was] all very real."

Eleanor believed that many of her symptoms, and her psychosis in particular, were caused by the medications that were injected into her. Her rendition of the events was that she initially got worse, and not better, and she attributed this both to the violence of the treatment she received—being involuntarily injected and "escorted" against her will to a seclusion room, where she was locked in—and to the effects of the medications, which made her thinking quite difficult and slowed. An alternative explanation—one that psychiatrists might prefer—would be that the mental illness made her agitated, disorganized, sleepless, intrusive, and delusionally paranoid; over the course of the first few days, the symptoms of the illness got progressively worse, but then with time, the medications made her better.

Eleanor's view that treatment caused her problems is not unique; as we discussed earlier, there is a growing antipsychiatry movement that contends that psychotropic medications are the cause of mental illness and that those who have had these treatments are survivors, not patients. Journalist Robert Whitaker, who wrote *Mad in America* and *Anatomy of an Epidemic*, has been quick to point out that as the use of psychiatric medications increased, so did the number of Americans who receive disability benefits for psychiatric illnesses. He believes that the medications are responsible for causing psychiatric disabilities.

Former NIMH director Dr. Thomas Insel has publicly stated that some individuals with schizophrenia do better with less medication over the long run, and schizophrenia researcher Dr. Nancy Andreasen has written that increased exposure to antipsychotic medications and increased numbers of psychotic episodes are *both* associated with brain atrophy or deterioration, creating a perplexing dilemma as to how aggressively people should be treated between episodes of psychosis. Antipsychiatry groups have speculated that the increased use of antidepressants has contributed to the rising suicide rates and even accounts for mass murders and other acts of violence.

Given these sentiments, it would be dismissive to simply write off Eleanor's belief that the medications caused her to be psychotic. People can certainly have very different responses to medications, and the distress is genuine even when the belief about causation is mistaken.

When this chicken-or-egg-first topic was broached with Eleanor, she replied:

For the patient, it is impossible to know what is causing the hallucinations and mental distortions. It is impossible to even know they are mental distortions and hallucinations while experiencing [them]. It seems like reality, which is why it is so terrifying. If the patient could realize the distortions are not reality, it would be much easier to deal with. In my case, I did not have the hallucinations before being injected, so I find it impossible to not consider multiple working hypotheses. It is a pretty amazing coincidence to pop into psychosis while getting out of the car at the emergency room, you have to admit. Prior to that, I just had slow, fuzzy, somewhat confused thinking. In the immediate aftermath of the injections, though, there was a terribly invasive effect on my brain. I am positive about the cause-[and]-effect of that because it started within minutes of injection. In my handwritten papers while [an] inpatient, I wrote that they were administering "the forgetting drug" because it seemed to wipe away all my memories of myself and who I am. I am guessing that was the Ativan. Hence, from my side, it is difficult to sort out, but that does not mean I do not think I was psychotic.

Initially, Eleanor was uncertain if her husband, Frank, would agree to be interviewed about what transpired during that time, but I found him to be surprisingly open. He said he wanted to help with this book so that others would not have to go through what his wife went through. Frank's memory was not as precise as Eleanor's. She said that her hospitalization had been a difficult situation for him as well: he had just returned to the United States, and he was busy caring for their pets and running her business while she was confined.

Frank recalled visiting Eleanor in the hospital: "It looked like she had recovered! That was the old Eleanor. I knew she was fine. She told me the medicines would wear off, and she'd feel normal, then they'd give them to her again."

Eleanor was upset with the day-to-day management of her care. The hospital initially had trouble accommodating her vegan diet, and she was under the impression that the staff considered her unconventional food preferences to be evidence that she was mentally ill. "I did not think they were trying to poison me per se, but I thought their persistent serving of meat to me was a plot, when it probably was incompetence and lack of concern."

Her husband was told he could bring food in for her, so Frank went to Whole Foods and bought lentil soup and other things Eleanor might like, but they were never prepared for her. At some point, Eleanor was given a vegetarian diet, and later she was seen by a nutritionist, who was able to obtain appropriate vegan food for her.

As she improved, Eleanor became aware that her behavior had been disruptive to others on the unit and that she had infringed on their rights. She had entered the rooms of other patients, and she had tried repeatedly to escape from the unit, once by pulling the fire alarm. On a different occasion, she hugged another patient; perhaps such an advance was not welcome.

"The other patients hated having me around when I was psychotic," Eleanor said. "I figured that out when I popped out of psychosis and discovered that all the patients were annoyed when I walked into the day-room, and they were impatient to get rid of me. I felt completely shunned when I first entered the dayroom in a nonpsychotic state."

While many things troubled Eleanor during her time in the hospital, she mentioned a few aspects she found helpful. One nurse drew her a bath and suggested she would find it relaxing. She did. And after she received privileges, she liked going outside with the smokers to be in the yard with trees and grass and fresh air, even though she was not a smoker. Eleanor also enjoyed the nightly visits with her husband and found them to be comforting.

Eleanor felt that many of the policies on the unit were demeaning. "If you wanted to ask a question, you had to stand at attention on a painted line opposite [the] nurses' station and wait your turn. They thought their paperwork was more important than our questions."

She did not like standing on a line to ask the nurses questions "at attention." I did not verify if such a rule existed, but assuming it did, I wonder if the nurses instituted this policy because they found it difficult to get their work done with patients approaching the nurses' station continually. While Eleanor perceived that the nurses would rather do their paperwork than attend to the patients, I might presume that the nurses received little pleasure from paperwork. It's not that I don't believe Eleanor's rendition of the events, but I like to play the devil's advocate, and as someone who has worked on hospital units, I can't help but wonder if there are other explanations aside from insensitivity, neglect, or malice. And of course, we could both be wrong; it's difficult to know the motives of other human beings unless they know and honestly tell us why they acted as they did.

In another example of disappointing care, Eleanor informed the staff that she was allergic to adhesive tape, a notation that was in every section of her chart where allergies were listed, and yet she said they still put adhesive tape on her at times. In general, she felt that her treatment was inconsiderate of her comfort and dismissive of her concerns. She felt her caretakers did not listen to her or strive to make her recovery a healing experience.

When asked what could have been different, Eleanor replied simply, "They could have been kinder."

As the days in the hospital went by, Eleanor got better. After September 11, there were no more episodes when she was placed in the seclusion room; on that day, she was noted to be "much less disorganized, less hyperverbal, less intrusive." She cooperated with the staff and took medications by mouth. But on September 12, the psychiatrist continued to note that "Patient is very paranoid, fixated on belief that night nurses want to kill her. She's a little less agitated this AM." While the notes overall reflect that she was less agitated, she remained "hyperverbal" and "hypomanic" throughout her hospitalization.

Dr. Ricki Pollycove, Eleanor's gynecologist, had commented to me, "She's always had this quality of having a mind that works faster than her speech, and sometimes it seems pressured." I wonder if that was what the staff saw as "hyperverbal" after the mania subsided. As two talkative people, Eleanor and I had no trouble filling hours with fast-paced conversation.

While Eleanor said her husband was initially relieved that she was hospitalized, by September 13, the unit social worker documented, "He questions whether patient needs to be in the hospital. Gave him feedback on patient's current behavior and he said he still believes it could be to patient's detriment to stay in the hospital."

In a family meeting on September 19, it was again documented that Frank felt that Eleanor could be managed outside the hospital. Eleanor remains angry that she was kept for days longer than was absolutely necessary, and she wondered if this was because there were empty beds on the unit and her insurance was paying most of the bill, while she and her husband paid the co-pays and other expenses that were not covered by her insurance.

Eleanor felt that she was held in the hospital too long and that once committed, there were no checks on the system to make sure she was released as soon as she no longer met the criteria for involuntary treatment. Psychiatrists—but not insurance companies—often want patients to remain in the hospital long enough to be certain they are really well enough to go home, but there are no studies on how long someone should be free of symptoms to allow for a safe discharge.

Eleanor felt that Frank's visits were instrumental in getting her to cooperate with the inpatient staff. On September 21, Eleanor was discharged to a partial hospitalization program, three weeks after being admitted to the inpatient unit. Dr. Green wrote in Eleanor's discharge note, "She was primarily treated for a psychiatric disorder, which seemed to be mania, which was acute and had been triggered by several family stressors over the previous months." He noted the changes in medication and put a final diagnosis of bipolar affective disorder, manic phase, and hypothyroidism.

Eleanor was discharged on the following daily psychiatric medications: Zyprexa, 25 mg; Abilify, 20 mg; Haldol, 10 mg; Cogentin, 2 mg; Klonopin, 1.5 mg. These are moderate to high doses of medications, three of which address psychosis. One reason Eleanor might have received such high doses of medications in unconventional combinations is because her symptoms were difficult to control, and hospitals are under pressure to release patients quickly. To contain difficult patients with more judicious use of medication requires a high staff-to-patient ratio, and most hospitals have been challenged to finance an optimal number of caretakers for very ill patients. But no psychiatrist would look at this unconventional combination of medications and be surprised to hear that Eleanor was sedated, felt drugged, and experienced side effects.

Eleanor concluded, "It sticks with you. I'm not sure I'll ever be fully over it. It's like child abuse. You could say that my father beat me, and I grew up to go to college and be a successful and responsible adult, but that doesn't make it okay, and it doesn't mean it goes away."

Eleanor's perception was that staff members were vindictive, inflicted pain as punishment, and played "mind games." Such treatment is not acceptable in any way, for any reason. There are unkind people in every profession, but they should be removed from patient care jobs. Being unkind is not a philosophy that is taught or condoned by the psychiatric profession.

Eleanor had been off medications for seven years when we spoke, and she had not had another psychotic episode. When I told this to Dr. Green, he stated, "She'll get sick again." I hope that Green's dismal prognosis for Eleanor will prove to be wrong, but only time will tell. In my own psychiatric practice, I often wish I had a crystal ball for such things.

After her discharge, Eleanor was able to return to school and then to work in a completely new field. She knows it is possible (or "not impossible," to use her words) that she might become sick again, but she tries to keep a handle on her stress level, and she makes sure to get enough sleep.

10

Ray DePaulo and Inpatient Psychiatry at a University Hospital

"I think we're committing some of the wrong people, for the wrong reasons, to the wrong places," said Dr. J. Raymond DePaulo Jr., the psychiatrist in chief at Johns Hopkins Hospital. "We should be committing patients who are severely mentally ill and can't take care of themselves, or people who are acutely suicidal and need protection and care. We should care for them in the hospital at least long enough to come up with a plan that helps them now and in the future. You know, you shouldn't need to be committed five times in your life."

In most large hospitals, even teaching hospitals, the department chair is an administrator who does not have the responsibility for running an inpatient service. At Johns Hopkins, the chair is like every other full-time faculty member in that he or she is required to spend a few months each year attending on an inpatient unit, teaching residents and medical students, conducting morning rounds, and being responsible for the day-to-day care of patients. DePaulo, who is also the Henry Phipps Professor and the director of the Department of Psychiatry and Behavioral Sciences, is no exception, and he takes his turn in the trenches willingly. This keeps his clinical skills sharp, and it allows for an appreciation of what it means to be a doctor on the wards, down to the details of listening to patients complain about the temperature of their food and the aggravation of trying to type a note into the electronic medical record.

DePaulo is slightly taller than average, slim, and earnest. He always wears a white lab coat when seeing patients. He is a serious man who wants to please, and he loves to talk about psychiatry. He's a natural teacher, and his enthusiasm is evident in bursts of nervous energy and a myriad of stories. DePaulo talks without a strong filter (in a good way) so if you want to know what's in his heart, you need only ask. The demands on his time are incessant; often he runs late and arrives flustered. If you phoned central casting and placed an order for an actor who was the perfect mix of the dignified professor and the distracted scientist, they might send someone much like DePaulo.

When I first mentioned this book to him, DePaulo agreed that it's a difficult situation when a family member wants to force a sick person to get care.

"I do everything I can to get patients to come in voluntarily. If the patient needs to be committed despite all my efforts, I do everything I can to protect their relationship with their loved ones who brought them for help. Even when a committed patient gets well, and even if he comes to agree that the hospitalization was necessary, he may never forgive the parent or spouse who initiated the commitment. Still, if you have to do it to save their life, then I tell the family, 'We have to do this.'"

DePaulo discussed the specific problems that face parents trying to help adult children who are ill: "It's interesting the conversations you have, and before we get to that step, I now script parents for these discussions. I tell them they need to go to their child and hold them close and say 'I can't lose you.' And if they cry genuine tears, so much the better. It is the truth and a difficult truth to tell your child who doesn't want to hear this."

He talked about how patients who have been committed—particularly people suffering from mania, which he specializes in—see their treatment after the fact. "Sometimes, they come to agree that they needed to be hospitalized, but in retrospect they say, 'It didn't have to be done *that way*,' and they talk about being brought in by the police, or being held down for emergency medications."

DePaulo noted that some patients never forgive a family member for negotiating their hospitalization, but psychiatrist Mark S. Komrad has had different experiences. Komrad writes in his book *You Need Help! A Step-by-Step Plan to Convince a Loved One to Get Counseling* about the aftermath of having a family member involuntarily hospitalized. In the chapter "How to Play Hardball," there is a section titled "Don't Be Intimidated by Fear of Damaging the Relationship." Komrad writes, "It is *remarkably common* for patients to completely change their hostile attitude toward their families after they get well. That hostility is often a by-product of the illness—the distorted thinking, the supercharged emotions, and the lack of insight into being sick—all of which can be expected to improve with treatment."

Once again, there are no data on patient responses to civil commitment, and psychiatrists are left with their own beliefs about what is in the best interests of the patient, which may depend on their own prior experiences.

Meyer 3 is just one floor of the psychiatry inpatient services at Johns Hopkins Hospital. There are 24 beds on the unit, covered by three separate teams, with each team responsible for the care of eight patients. The permanent staff includes the unit clerks, nurses, occupational therapists, social workers, aides, and housekeepers. The nonpermanent staff includes the attending physicians (senior psychiatrists who take turns rotating onto the floors for a month at a time); resident psychiatrists in training, who stay on a service for three months; any number of students, who are there for days to weeks; and security guards, who come to the floor when they are needed, often just for a few hours at a time.

The entrance to Meyer 3 is by an elevator, which opens to an enclosed area across from the nurses' station. When the unit clerk saw me pulling on the locked door, she pressed a buzzer to let me in. Mornings on the unit were a bustle of activity. There was a large, open area, lined with windows, which served as a living space. A flat-screen TV held the attention of a handful of patients, some dressed in jeans, others in hospital-issue gowns. The patients who would be getting electroconvulsive treatments later in the morning were tethered to intravenous lines dripping clear fluid. The dining area was filled with patients; staff and security watched over them or ate something themselves (or did both). A nurse sat off to the side, entering data into one of many computers on the unit. There were large, mobile computers and a number of pull-down computers built into the walls. Medicines were dispensed, the doctors and medical students gathered for rounds, and despite all that went on, the unit was surprisingly orderly.

I visited Meyer 3 for a week in February 2014. Rounds began at 8:30 a.m. in the office of the psychiatry resident. When DePaulo entered, the resident relinquished her desk with the Hopkins computer and moved to a chair with her own laptop. There was also a medical student, a social worker, an occupational therapist—all with laptops—and a nurse, who came with one of the large movable computer stations that I later heard someone refer to as "the cow," or computer on wheels.

The nurse discussed a patient while everyone typed. They went around the room, taking turns adding their observations of each patient from their own discipline's perspective: topics included a patient's symptoms; medications; the management of any medical conditions; what he had done the day before; how she'd slept; who visited; what activities she participated in; and how he reported feeling. They planned for follow-up after the hospitalization as well. The discussions included everything from how the patient's utility bills were getting paid during the stay to whether she might eventually benefit from owning a dog to how another would cope with baking cookies in occupational therapy while on a diabetic diet.

It was also the time for the team to discuss patients' legal status as voluntary or involuntary, and if they had required the use of restraints, seclusion, or intramuscular injections of medications over the course of the previous day. After all the talk among the professionals, each patient was brought into the room.

DePaulo took over from there. Patient by patient, he asked how they were. He told them what the team members had said, giving the patient a chance to confirm, deny, or elaborate. One patient complained every day about the taste of his medication, and it became a bit of a joke, a lighthearted way for DePaulo to connect with him. The psychiatrist acknowledged the patient's distress over the taste as he reviewed why this particular medication was necessary compared to the alternatives.

DePaulo often asked the patients if things were going okay on the unit, and that's when he heard that the food was not being served at the right temperature. At the end of each session, he asked the patient if he or she had questions for the team, and he often asked the team members if they had more questions for the patient. A treatment plan was set. One gentleman bargained; he wanted to be discharged on Saturday, but DePaulo wanted him to wait until Monday, and he explained why. The encounters were brief, the setting lacked intimacy, the keyboards chattered away, but the interaction was thoughtful and certainly not adversarial.

For the short time each patient was in the office with the team, DePaulo tried to make some connection. He'd single something out and comment on it.

"Like, you're seeing things in the corner of your eye, just as you're about to fade off to sleep?" he asked one patient, who was discussing her difficult nights and an odd sense that she might be hallucinating. A flash of recognition came across her face, as if to say that yes, he'd gotten it, he understood exactly what she was going through. He reassured her those weren't real hallucinations, that seeing or imagining things only in that period just before sleep was not something to be concerned about.

With another patient, DePaulo struggled to connect; nothing quite did it. It was obvious he was trying, but the patient was just not in a place for much more than yes or no answers. When she left, I broke from my role as the observer.

"The patient made you anxious," I said.

He could have been annoyed or defensive, but DePaulo responded with openness. "She did make me anxious. It doesn't take much."

When the last patient left, the team went to visit those who could not come to the office. The first stop was the room of a woman who was feeling too ill to get out of bed. DePaulo asked her a few questions.

While psychiatrists typically do not share much about their personal lives with patients, DePaulo sometimes strayed from that standard, at least briefly. This patient, who suffered from sciatica, was rubbing the front of her leg.

"Does it hurt there?" he asked.

"No, in back."

"Yes, when I had sciatica it hurt on the back and side of my leg."

DePaulo put the Freudian image of the psychiatrist as a "blank slate" aside, trading it for the kind, caring doctor with a hefty dose of shared humanity. For a field that has struggled with being seen as overly paternalistic or as all about pushing pills, this was not a bad thing.

Rounds lasted roughly three hours. All eight patients were seen when possible, and we reconvened later in the afternoon to go over any major changes that had occurred during the day.

I should mention that I hesitated to use Johns Hopkins Hospital as a setting to write about inpatient psychiatry. Its Department of Psychiatry is consistently named as one of the top five departments in the country in *US News and World Report*'s hospital rankings. Does it indicate anything about inpatient psychiatry in the United States to say that all is well at the nation's few top hospitals: that the doctors are kind and thoughtful; that the seclusion rooms are mostly empty; that the only involuntary patient I observed was afforded the luxury of having three security guards with him at all times, a measure that kept him and everyone else on the unit safe while minimizing (but not eliminating) the need to restrain, seclude, or repeatedly inject him with medications he might refuse to take orally? Does it help that I learned weeks later that the same patient still managed to rip the flat-screen television from the dayroom wall? The staff-to-patient ratio was high, and every effort was made to address patient concerns. Not one of the patients I saw was having the same experience as Eleanor reported.

The truth is that Johns Hopkins was not my first choice; I was there because they would have me. I first tried a community hospital near my home, which has a single psychiatric floor. I had worked in the outpatient department years before, and I remain fond of the chairman. The parking was easier and the commute shorter. The hospital has a good reputation, but it is community care, not a major teaching institution and not a department that garners enough interest for national rankings.

When I explained that I wanted to shadow an inpatient doctor and maybe someone in the Emergency Department, I was told quite courteously that I couldn't use their patients for my book. Federal privacy regulations, known as HIPAA, require that patients authorize others to have access to any of their personal health information. If that wasn't touchy enough, I wanted to observe civilly committed patients, those who are so mentally ill as to be dangerous and in need of involuntary care; the issue of the capacity to consent was quite sticky.

It soon became clear that it didn't matter who I was, who I knew, or how noble a project this book might be. Observing psychiatric patients in a role outside of treatment or education was going to be a problem. I changed tactics and tried another hospital: I asked to observe a psychiatrist and said I would not be writing about the patients. But this still required that I be present in the treatment setting and able to eavesdrop on the interactions, and again my request was denied.

I thought it might be easier at Hopkins because I hold an appointment there, and until recently I had worked in the Community Psychiatry Program on the first floor of the Meyer Building. I had trained on Meyer 3 as a resident in 1989–1990, and I sometimes visited my clinic patients on the unit and went on rounds when they were in the hospital. I had a key, I had an ID, and I had the enthusiastic support of Dr. DePaulo.

When I first asked, in July 2013, I was told that a clinical director had to be consulted. When I didn't hear back, I tried again and was told the legal department needed to be consulted. Months went by. When finally I contacted DePaulo, he apologized for taking so long to respond—he had been attending on a unit—so I asked if I could write about *him*. He was kind and gregarious; he is proud of his department and feels it is important to showcase the good work that gets done at Hopkins. While others avoided my calls or told me to take my project elsewhere, DePaulo's response to my request to shadow him on an inpatient unit was quick and welcoming.

I came to the unit two days later and was met with instructions for paperwork. I needed to read and sign a HIPAA form. DePaulo needed to talk with every patient on the service and ask their permission for a visitor to join the already-crowded rounds, and the patients needed to sign a release. I could not stay in rounds for any patient who objected; none did. I had to agree not to release any personal health information and to allow my writing to be seen by the department before publication. I agreed. As I thought about it, I realized that there are few nonfiction books set on psychiatric units, although patients are not legally prevented from writing about their experiences. This leaves the public with what's garnered from movies, and inpatient psychiatry is still best known for Nurse Ratched in *One Flew over the Cuckoo's Nest*. It's a hidden world, open only to those who are in enough despair to gain admittance. Visitors get a glimpse during stipulated hours. No wonder there is so much mystery and hesitation.

During the week I came for rounds, Meyer 3 was fairly quiet. I checked the seclusion room every day—it was always empty. It was a small room with a bare mattress on the floor and two doors. One opened to the back of the nurses' station, the other to the hallway where the patient rooms were located. A handwritten sign over the door in the hallway read "Relaxation Room." I wasn't sure if that would be considered humor by someone being escorted in against their will. The walls were painted a shade of blue, and there were a few notable chips in the paint, likely from someone's banging.

DePaulo has been psychiatrist in chief at Johns Hopkins Hospital since 2002. He talked about his predecessor, Paul McHugh.

When Paul McHugh came here as chairman back in 1975, there were people being put into seclusion, and no one was watching them. And Paul said he didn't want seclusion being used as a substitute for manpower. He insisted that whenever anyone was put into seclusion, he wanted a nurse sitting outside the door, watching, and it changed everything. That wasn't true of most hospitals. In a hospital, if you don't continue to ask questions and renew efforts and make things better—if you're just going to leave things the way they are and let them be—that leads to corruption.

During one morning report, we heard that a patient had required a great deal of care. He had a long history of illness and violence, and on that occasion he was agitated to the point of needing first an oral medication to calm him and, when that didn't work, an injection.

Many patients' civil rights advocates say that it would be natural to be agitated in these restrictive settings, and they claim that the insensitivity and intrusiveness of staff provoke understandable distress. Psychiatry's response, they contend, is to exert control where understanding, kindness, and freedom would take care of the problem.

I was impressed that the Meyer 3 team reviewed the incident with that particular patient in its full context. The patient had been provoked by another patient, who took a personal item belonging to him. He became distraught, was given oral medication, and later received an injection. The instigating patient, who had taken the item and provoked the event, was discharged from the unit. The situation was rectified, and the staff discussed ways to prevent this from happening again.

"Did he get it back?" DePaulo asked about the item in question.

"Yes, we found it in the laundry room," a nurse replied.

I am not saying that mistakes and miscommunications never happen, but in my years as a psychiatrist, I have never witnessed the vindictiveness that Eleanor described, nor the unabashed contempt that Dr. Julie Holland confessed to in her memoir, *Weekends at Bellevue*.

Four floors of the Meyer Building are devoted to inpatient psychiatry, a total of 96 beds. Insurance companies are not eager to pay the $2,500 per day cost for the hospital, and many privately insured patients have high co-payments. Insurers demand justification for each hospital day. This means that all patients in the hospital are quite ill, and many are quite dangerous, since preauthorization is typically denied for any patient who is not deemed to be high risk. "Medical necessity" criteria select for those in danger, and psychiatry is the only specialty where insurers set the bar for admission to be a life-threatening level of illness. If the illness is not actually life-threatening, then the patient is usually asserting that he feels suicidal and can't promise not to harm himself.

Psychiatry is not inexpensive under the best of circumstances, and in cases where the patient requires one-on-one, around-the-clock supervision, expensive medications, and highly personalized care, the costs can be exorbitant. At the same time, Johns Hopkins is located in East Baltimore—a neighborhood with rampant poverty, crime, and addiction—and many of the patients are on Medicaid and juggling financial stresses, social isolation, medical and mental illnesses, and substance abuse problems. Nothing about it is easy.

I asked to sit in on the civil commitment hearings—with patient consent, of course. They still happen on Wednesdays just as they did when I was a resident, and the same attending psychiatrist remained in charge. During my observation week, I was told there would be no hearings that Wednesday because every patient who had been certified from the Emergency Department had signed in, changing their status from involuntary to voluntary.

There were several patients on Meyer 3 who had been admitted on certificates, who then agreed to sign in on a voluntary basis. I asked DePaulo if he would ask one man why he made that decision. The patient responded, "They talk to me with love and respect, and I feel comfortable."

In the battle over involuntary psychiatric care, DePaulo is not one of the stakeholders; he's a mood disorders researcher and a department administrator. He's not out there advocating for legislation to either narrow or broaden the criteria to get patients into the hospital against their will. His thoughts about involuntary treatment revolve around what's best for his patients and for his department, and some of that is about finances and impediments to offering high-quality care.

"You can't quite make this all fit into looking at involuntary admissions. It's really about looking at the system of care, with 'certs' being one of the ways we can misappropriate resources. . . . ED docs are afraid of psychiatric patients. And they're afraid of suicidal patients. If a patient threatens suicide and they won't take it back persuasively, they get admitted."

DePaulo went on to talk about patients who are admitted involuntarily because they don't have the capacity to consent because of intellectual disabilities, including mental retardation. "What typically happens is that there will be a new staff member in a group home, a fuss ensues, and a patient throws a glass. They end up in the hospital for months."

He noted that these are patients who may have once been sent to state hospitals, "but the state hospitals are now for the courts, and the psychiatrists didn't get a voice."

In Maryland—as in many states—the majority of state hospital beds are now used for forensic patients, those who have either been found legally insane following a crime, or those who are too ill to stand trial for an alleged criminal act and are getting treatment to restore their competency. Some patients are transferred to state hospitals when they are too violent to be managed in a private hospital. In addition, the Emergency Medical Treatment and Active Labor Act mandated that hospitals with empty beds must accept patients in transfer from other Emergency Departments. All these forces have collided to make hospital beds, which have decreased in number over time, a coveted commodity.

"I don't see communication across the lines so that we actually get people the help they need," DePaulo said.

> Here's the thing: we're not getting people to the right place. We have the blind men and the elephant approach to medicine, and everybody knows that. So you have a hearing, and there's someone in charge of letting people out of the hospital if they are there inappropriately, but that person is not in charge of making sure they get care and don't end up walking in front of traffic later. The patients we have on the floors now, as opposed to way back when, maybe 1980, . . . they are much more often now people with drug and personality and behavior problems, and they have long records of conduct issues. A much smaller percentage are the chronically and severely mentally ill. I think it's because this is how society is allocating resources. This is just an estimate, but maybe 25 percent of patients who are committed are psychotic and disorganized. I'm frustrated with how we use our resources, and it's not just about being efficient, it's about being effective. I want us to get the right kind of care to people.

I mentioned that things were fairly calm and orderly when I was on the unit.

"You happened to be there at a calm time. If there was one more patient who needed a lot, it would be different. We had one patient taking up half the resources," he said, referring to the gentleman who had three security guards watching him. "When there's a second one on the unit doing that, things change."

Dr. DePaulo was kind enough to let me observe him deliver care in an inner-city teaching hospital where the Department of Psychiatry is a single cog in a large institution that delivers the full spectrum of medical care. This was the same type of hospital that Lily was in, and it represents only one kind of inpatient experience. Eleanor, however, had been treated at a free-standing private psychiatric facility, the topic of our next chapter.

Steven Sharfstein, Bruce Hershfield, and Free-Standing Psychiatric Hospitals

The exit from the parking garage at Johns Hopkins Hospital dumps a visitor into the heart of East Baltimore. The hospital itself is an enormous complex of buildings topped by an iconic dome. Venturing just a few blocks away, the reality of the streets becomes apparent. There are boarded-up row homes, young men sitting idle on stoops in the middle of the day, children making their way to and from school. Boxes with blue flashing lights—police surveillance cameras—loom from the telephone poles with an intense intrusiveness, perched like giant birds' nests. Motorists make their way across the Orleans Street bridge to the middle of town and Charles Street. From there, the drive uptown is a colorful one, and with each click of the odometer, the real estate gets a little pricier. The street is lined first by stores and brownstones, then by row houses, and finally by softer suburban areas with large, gracious, landscaped homes.

Outside the city limits, there is a country club on one side of Charles Street, and a few minutes later, one comes to Sheppard Pratt Health System, another large psychiatric facility. Until about 15 years ago, the road to enter the hospital grounds passed right through the gatehouse, a curiosity that amused children and led visitors into a beautiful, sprawling campus. Now, the road swerves around the house; it was moved to ensure the stability of the aging, historic landmark. Construction projects have added a new hospital and a conference center, and the once beautiful grounds now provide more services and more functionality. In past generations, some of the hospital's 400 acres were used to grow corn and pumpkins.

Now, part of the original grounds is leased to a local university, and college dorms line one edge of the hospital campus.

Traditionally, psychiatric care in the United States has been determined by the patient's wallet. People who go to the Emergency Department of a university or to a community hospital are admitted if there are beds. If there are no available beds, the patient is transferred to another facility. For those with private health insurance, this might be a private psychiatric hospital. For those with no insurance, state hospitals have provided care. Because private insurance historically had limits, those with long-term chronic illnesses often found their way to state hospitals as well.

The beds in Maryland's state hospital system are now being used for the evaluation and treatment of people charged with crimes or found legally insane, rather than for merely indigent patients. This is true in many other states as well. The traditional public-private divide has been blurred. Sheppard Pratt used to be one of the private hospitals—a place where people stayed to heal, and the rolling green lawns of the campus were dotted with Adirondack chairs.

I found Dr. Steven Sharfstein in his office, a large room busy with books, papers, photographs of famous people, diplomas, and awards. Sharfstein is the president and chief executive officer of Sheppard Pratt Health System and a former president of the American Psychiatric Association. If Dr. DePaulo's uniform is his white lab coat, then Dr. Sharfstein's uniform is his dark suit. He is a quiet and thoughtful man, but it doesn't take much effort to get him talking about his ideas and plans for the future. Sheppard Pratt, like Johns Hopkins, is consistently ranked as one of the top psychiatric facilities in the country by *US News and World Report*.

Sharfstein is an influential man, and he has strong feelings about involuntary psychiatric treatments. He has been a NAMI member since 1979, and he went to Annapolis in 2014 to testify in favor of legislation that would allow for the involuntary treatment of patients outside of hospitals. "I have a public health perspective," he said.

> I've worked in jails, and the fact is that people with schizophrenia, with comorbid substance use, and with affective [mood] disorders are in the street, and they end up in jail. It's a public health disaster of the first degree. People are dying, and people are being abused. We have to be aggressive about getting people out of jails and into treatment. The Cook

County Jail, the LA County Jail, and Rikers Island are the biggest mental health facilities in the country. The psychiatric patients are in with the general population, and they are being victimized. I get one or two calls a week from people with mentally ill family members; they are at wit's end and can't get help. I think in the face of the consequences of not getting treatment, which are potentially devastating, if not life-threatening, there should be a way of getting people care even against their will. Ultimately, forced care is an alternative to criminalization.

His sentiments mirrored those of Fuller Torrey and the Treatment Advocacy Center.

At one time, Sheppard Pratt treated patients with means, those with insurance or the resources to pay, and patients stayed for months, if not longer. Now, the hospital still treats privately insured patients, but it also takes those with Medicaid and Medicare and the uninsured, a result of the fact that Maryland contracts with community facilities to provide beds for those who formerly were treated in the state hospital system. In many ways, this is an equalizer: the poor and uninsured get the same care as the wealthy.

The new 280-bed hospital has an average length of stay of approximately 10 days, and there are 200 admissions per week. But psychiatric medications often take weeks to work, the first choice of medication often doesn't work or requires augmentation, and psychotherapy is a process that takes time. With such short lengths of stay, some patients do not get optimal care.

Many patients are initially admitted involuntarily. As is true at Hopkins, only a small percentage of those patients go to a hearing; the rest sign in voluntarily. The hospital usually conducts three to six civil commitment hearings a week. It is this type of free-standing psychiatric hospital where Eleanor received treatment in Northern California.

Sharfstein has overseen the Sheppard Pratt Health System since 1986. He talked about the evolution of care during this time.

"When I came, the average length of stay was 80 days. Ninety percent of our patients had private insurance. Since then, the purpose of hospitals has changed; back then, you stayed until you got better or until you ran out of insurance. Now, people come in to be stabilized, and most care is given on an outpatient basis. It was thought, then, that if a person was admitted for two weeks, then it was inappropriate because that was not long enough to treat them."

"I'm a community psychiatrist," Sharfstein noted, "and I feel strongly that hospitals should be for short-term care with most care being given near where people live and work."

Sheppard's new hospital was built in 2005, and it connects to the older, historic building, which still houses patients. The units are arranged as spokes; hallways branch from a central nursing station at the hub. It has a state-of-the-art feel. We entered a unit that treats patients with psychosis and were greeted by a large man in uniform, who was sitting on a chair by the door.

"We have 'milieu officers,'" Sharfstein explained. "They are mental health professionals dressed in uniform, unarmed, because we have more aggressive patients now. In 1986, when I came here, aggressive patients were rare. But now, if you try to set limits, people may strike out, and we're trying to keep our units as safe as possible; we've had some bad assaults."

The officer explains the unit rules to new patients, and he is trained to spot trouble and de-escalate situations before things get out of control.

Sharfstein said that the patient rooms are all private, and each has its own bathroom. "It's about maintaining dignity and respect, but it's an issue with suicidal patients. People are less likely to attempt suicide when there's a roommate." He noted that there have been some serious attempts, and two patients have died of suicide in the hospital over the past 20 years.

I wanted to look at one last hospital setting: a traditional state hospital. Neither Eleanor nor Lily was ever treated at that type of institution, but in the mid-twentieth century, state hospitals housed hundreds of thousands of people in the United States. These facilities traditionally provided care for those who had no insurance and for those who needed long-term, often custodial, care because they didn't get better.

If you exit Sheppard Pratt on Charles Street, then take the Baltimore Beltway west to Liberty Road and drive a dozen or so miles to Sykesville, a more rural part of Maryland, you'll come to the Springfield Hospital Center, which opened in July 1896 on land that was once a family farm and estate. The campus is a collection of brick buildings, sprawled over hundreds of acres. At one time, the hospital farm made a profit; the patients grew enough food to feed the hospital community and sell what remained. The baseball field is still used for patient-staff games, and the cemetery, which last accepted admissions in 1961, has fresh flowers adorning its mass name plaque. At the top of the hill, by the house that was once the superintendent's residence, is a single gravesite dedicated to all who have donated their bodies for medical education in the state of Maryland.

The original hospital building is a beautiful Georgian brick structure with a cupola. Today, it is used by the state police as a training center. Some of the other buildings are boarded up, and at one end of the campus there is a semicircle of abandoned brick buildings. These once contained the epilepsy colony, but they now remain a haunted village of abandoned decay. This is a historical site, so they can't be demolished.

At its peak in the 1950s, Springfield housed more than 3,000 patients, some for decades. Currently, the census runs about 230, split among 11 units; a few of the patients have lived there for many years. This decrease in long-term residents mirrors the national trend: we now have less than 10 percent of the state hospital beds we once had, while the US population has doubled. Certainly, many people were held in state hospitals for far too long when they would have done well in the community. But some of the beds have been eliminated at a human cost. There is nowhere to house people who are chronically ill or chronically addicted, and some of these people end up living on the streets or in jails and prisons. And worse, there are not enough beds for those who are acutely ill. Our confidence in medications to treat mental disorders on an outpatient basis has been overextended.

For the most part, admission to Springfield Hospital Center now comes through the court system. People are sent there if they are charged with a crime but are too ill to stand trial. They are treated to restore their competency so the judicial process can move forward. Others have been declared "not criminally responsible" for a crime they've been found guilty of committing, and they are sent to Springfield to recover. After these patients are treated, they may be released to the community on "conditional release," a status similar to being paroled. If they become ill again, they can be readmitted to Springfield for treatment, and this admission may be on a voluntary basis without the intervention of the courts.

Patients who have been found insane or incompetent to stand trial are admitted involuntarily through a process known as criminal (as opposed to civil) commitment, because it is authorized through Maryland's criminal procedure laws. If there are no hospital beds available, they wait in jail. Some people are sent to the hospital for treatment that can't be administered in jail. For example, a patient who is deemed to need a court order for long-term involuntary medication would be transferred to Springfield for a hearing on this issue since Maryland law does not allow medication hearings to take place in jail. Still others are sent by a mental health court as an alternative to remaining in a correctional facility. Maryland's maximum security forensic hospital is reserved for the more violent patients, so many of those in Springfield are there for trespassing, indecent exposure, disturbing the peace, resisting arrest, minor assault, and any number of other crimes that resulted from their compromised mental states. There are still patients in the state hospital on civil, as opposed to criminal, commitment, but the push has been to move acute care to community hospitals.

Dr. Brian Hepburn was the executive director of Maryland's Department of Health and Mental Hygiene at the time we communicated, and he elaborated on the changes in who is admitted to state hospitals.

> We started the original change in 2002 with the central region of the state and completed the change statewide in 2010 with the Eastern Shore. Previously, if an uninsured person went to an Emergency Department with an inpatient psychiatric unit, the person was admitted to that hospital's inpatient unit. Uninsured persons who went to the Emergency Department of hospitals without an inpatient psychiatric unit were sent to the state hospitals. The decision to admit from the ED to a state hospital prior to 2002–2010 was based primarily on the person being uninsured. It is interesting that the public hospitals for the uninsured for physical health care stopped in Maryland in the mid-[19]70s to early '80s, due to the all-payer system, but it took until the 2000s for mental health to catch up. The idea of the all-payer system was that everyone should get the same care regardless of ability to pay.

The state began paying private psychiatric hospitals to accept those without insurance, instead of sending them to the state hospitals. Hepburn noted a 70 percent decrease in the admission rate to state hospitals over the 10-year period ending in 2012.

"We do occasionally transfer patients from other hospitals," he said, "but not based on length of time and not for the convenience of the hospital.

There are still people in the state hospitals who stay months if they need that level of care."

The long-term units were clean but institutional, similar to schools built in the 1960s, with tile and cinder block walls, linoleum floors, and fluorescent lighting. During my visit, the patients lingered in the halls, waiting to go to groups, and boredom hung in the air. The building included a small gym with basketball hoops, a volleyball net, and some aerobic machines. A brick courtyard was fully enclosed, but it was too cold and rainy on the day I was there for anyone to want to be outside. The dining area seated people at round tables of four. Some of the bedrooms were private, but others held as many as four people, with the beds separated by floor-to-ceiling hospital curtains for privacy. A seclusion room was empty, and a nurse estimated that no one had been placed in it for the previous month.

The acute units, also called "admission" units, were in newer buildings with vaulted ceilings and more natural light. The seclusion room there was also empty, but a staff member noted that one patient had been in and out, most recently five days before. The campus was so large that buses transported people from one building to another, and select patients could work at coveted jobs at the canteen or print shop.

Dr. Bruce Hershfield was the superintendent at Springfield from 1986 to 1993, at a time when the patients were people who either had no health insurance or had used up their benefits. He recalled that when he started, the hospital had more than 1,000 patients. By the time he left, the census was under 400.

"When I got there, people were sleeping on mattresses on the floor because they weren't discharging people fast enough. I had them bring up beds so that at least everyone would have their own bed. They got them from the basement, the original beds from 1896."

Hershfield, who now has a private practice and is a former speaker of the American Psychiatric Association assembly, said about the patients who were in the hospital involuntarily: "The committed patients didn't want to be there. They often wouldn't take medication. And the staff were afraid of the patients because they kept getting assaulted. What helped? We got the [drinks containing] caffeine out of the Coke machine, and we could show that the violence went down. People were getting jacked up by drinking six Cokes at a time."

Hershfield talked about involuntary commitment and suicidal patients.

"Most of the time, people were committed who wouldn't have killed themselves; that's pretty clear. But some of the time, they would, and it's too dangerous. You could spend your whole career in a courtroom for malpractice hearings if you're wrong even occasionally." Hershfield was echoing DePaulo's sentiment that doctors are afraid to release suicidal patients from Emergency Departments.

"You have to be careful. In private practice, I can keep people out of the hospital. I meet with them on the weekends if need be. It's cost-effective to avoid hospitalizing people, and sometimes the hospital can be traumatizing and the other patients can be violent or upsetting. And I think people like to be able to say they've never been in a hospital."

Hershfield shared his thoughts on legislation that would make it easier to commit people. "I don't think it's a good idea. Does the state have an obligation to put someone in a place they don't want to be because they don't like their beliefs? If someone's dangerous and we need to protect them or the citizenry, I can see that."

Even within the mainstream psychiatric community, we don't always agree on what's best for our patients, what's best for society, and what the standard for involuntary hospitalization should be. We likely capture many patients who don't need hospitalization in the name of being on the safe side or based on worry about the possibility of bad outcomes. And even with involuntary hospitalization as an option, we still miss 40,000 people a year who die by suicide and perhaps another 1,000 who commit homicide.

Annette Hanson and the Use of Seclusion and Restraint

Eleanor talked quite a bit about her time in seclusion. The staff sometimes turned off the light, and the light was connected to the room's fan, so she became uncomfortable in the dark with the stale air. Feeling like she might suffocate, she lay on the floor and tried to get air by putting her lips to the crack under the door. Eleanor reported that she still gets flashbacks when she's in closed spaces. The hospitalization was a very difficult time, and Eleanor wanted comfort, not isolation. At the same time, her behavior was disorganized and intrusive; she was bothering the other patients. Would it have sufficed to assign a one-on-one aide to help her? We can't really know if it was necessary to place Eleanor in seclusion.

As noted earlier, Lily cooperated with her caregivers for the most part and was never placed in a seclusion room. Neither woman was ever held in physical restraints, a practice that is no longer considered to be therapeutic and is used only to ensure safety. The use of physical restraints is now carefully regulated and is much less frequent than in the past.

For the discussion that follows in this chapter, we change narrators. While Dr. Miller conducted the interviews in the rest of the book, this story belongs to Dr. Hanson.

The Clifton T. Perkins Hospital Center is a state psychiatric facility, but unlike most state hospitals it is designated specifically as a "forensic" hospital. This means that the hospital is designed to be a secure facility in order to treat people charged with serious crimes or people who have been adjudicated legally insane for a serious offense. Unlike the situation in most psychiatric hospitals, patients may be admitted to a forensic hospital indefinitely—sometimes for years—until a court determines that they are either no longer mentally ill or no longer dangerous. Forensic hospitals care for patients who are criminal defendants, but may also manage care for patients who are too violent to be treated in a nonsecure psychiatric hospital.

A doctor in a forensic hospital has one of two roles with a patient. She could be the treating physician, or she could be the doctor designated to perform a court-ordered evaluation to determine legal sanity or to determine competence to stand trial. As a forensic training director, my role is to teach psychiatrists how to do competency and sanity evaluations. My story begins on a medium-security ward, where I had gone to review a defendant's chart for an evaluation.

I didn't see the attack coming. I had noticed the patient standing near the door of the inpatient unit, shifting anxiously from foot to foot. He was staring at me with a blank expression. I recognized that expression as a "negative symptom," a sign of schizophrenia that's common in someone with a serious psychotic illness.

As I left the nursing station, he walked toward me as if to say hello or to ask a question. But instead, the patient raised his fist and punched me across the temple. My glasses flew off, and my head whipped sideways.

I called for help. Nurses and security technicians ran to form a human shield between me and the patient. Seeing this, the patient lowered his fist and calmly walked away. Within moments, someone was handing me a cold compress to put on my face. I found out much later that the patient had assaulted a nurse in the medical clinic earlier that day.

After the incident, I was sent to the Human Resources Department to complete the required post-assault paperwork. I filled out an incident report, provided information for the hospital insurance carrier, and was given a referral to the employee health clinic in case I needed medical care. Only after the paperwork was done did I have time to reflect. I wondered what happened to the patient; I appreciated the immediate and professional response by the nursing staff. I knew this was a reflection of both their experience and their annual hospital training.

As a forensic psychiatrist, I've spent a couple of decades working with violent people in a maximum security prison and in a forensic hospital. This sounds like dangerous work, but in fact I had never been assaulted until then. The event left me a bit shaken for the rest of the day. My colleagues were concerned and supportive.

"It's happened to all of us," one of them said to me.

I was invited to attend a co-worker support group, an activity sponsored by the hospital to assist employees who had been assaulted on the job.

I wasn't seriously injured. Some mental health workers haven't been as fortunate. Psychiatrists have suffered facial fractures and brain injuries from patient assaults, and some have even been killed. That day, I was one of the lucky ones. Caring for very sick people involves carefully balancing on a tightrope between respecting the patient's freedom and autonomy, and protecting others from harm. As we've seen in previous chapters, taking away someone's freedom and admitting that person to a psychiatric unit against her or his will may be traumatic and upsetting. The fear, discomfort, and embarrassment that goes along with the use of physical restraints or placement in a seclusion room adds another layer of trauma that may deter people from seeking care in the future or from disclosing symptoms even to a trusted mental health professional. Psychiatrists try to avoid the use of these interventions, even in a forensic hospital.

But psychiatrists also have a competing obligation to safeguard the rights and privileges of other patients and the staff members on the psychiatric unit. People who are so ill that they run through the halls screaming, or repeatedly disrupt the treatment team by making calls to police from the unit, or who—in a worst case scenario—become assaultive to other patients, staff, or visitors create a dilemma for psychiatrists. In one survey of day hospital patients, one-quarter of them reported that they had been assaulted by another patient during a previous hospitalization.

Clearly, this kind of inpatient environment would be upsetting to live in and could hardly be considered therapeutic. When one patient's symptoms infringe on the rights of others, the psychiatrist is forced to make a difficult choice between patient safety and patient freedom.

The move to reduce the use of seclusion and restraint started with a series of newspaper articles entitled "Deadly Restraint" published in the *Hartford Courant* in 1998. The five-part series published interviews with formerly restrained patients, like 36-year-old Tina Puziello, who described her experience while hospitalized in the late 1980s and early 1990s:

I said I wanted to go to the other side of the building. I wanted to go to that side because I wanted to have a cigarette and a cup of coffee or whatever. I did that a couple of times. I was pretty soft-spoken and very depressed, but after a while of asking to go to the other side, I became frustrated and I banged on the window and I said I wanted to leave. I raised my voice and I have a loud voice.

I guess it frightened them and the fact that I yelled and punched the door. I guess they thought I was out of control. I heard them call a code—"Dr. Strong"—and about eight guys came and put me in this thing. It could have been five or six. It was scary.

They didn't throw me on the floor on my face, thank God. They used the other way: where everybody took a limb and then they picked me up and put me into the body bag.

It was like a straitjacket except that it was like a canvas material, a green color canvas. I believe my hands were in front. There are long sleeves and everything and then it has loops and ties that go all the way down from your neck. Like putting a shirt on that's too long and then they tie the ends of the shirt. Your hands are in there and then the whole thing is tightened.

As you wiggle around, they are tightening it more. They tie it all the way down. It went all the way down to your ankles. I guess they called it a body bag because it covers your whole body. Then it's easy for them to lift you. You're like a mummy, except your head isn't wrapped.

Following the restraint-related death of an 11-year-old boy in a Connecticut psychiatric hospital, the newspaper surveyed mental health facilities for the developmentally disabled and group homes in all 50 states, and discovered there had been 142 deaths in the previous decade, during or shortly after seclusion and restraint. One-quarter of the people who died were children, one as young as 6 years old, and seven people were in their seventies. One-third of the deaths were due to asphyxiation, some caused by actions that were clearly inappropriate and unrelated to the use of medically approved hospital restraints, such as a 16-year-old boy who died because a towel was wrapped around his mouth. Patients died due to inadequate staff training in the use of restraints and because the restrained patients were not monitored for breathing or circulation problems. Some were restrained face-down, a practice that has long been known to cause suffocation.

The *Courant* reported that the actual death rates from restraints in psychiatric units were unknown because accrediting agencies and the federal government didn't collect that data. Only one state, New York, even had a requirement for private and state facilities to report deaths. Few deaths were investigated, and no one was prosecuted. The facilities where the deaths occurred remained open to admissions.

In 1980, Congress passed the Mental Health Systems Act, which established a federal Patient Bill of Rights. This law required psychiatric units and behavioral health facilities to ensure that patients have "the right to freedom from restraint or seclusion, other than as a mode or course of treatment or restraint or seclusion during an emergency situation if such restraint or seclusion is pursuant to or documented contemporaneously by the written order of a responsible mental health professional." The law also required "the right to a humane treatment environment that affords reasonable protection from harm and appropriate privacy to such person with regard to personal needs."

But who decides what a "humane treatment environment" should be or what constitutes an "emergency situation"? When is restraint and seclusion "a mode or course of treatment" versus a punitive or vindictive act, or just a lazy person's way to quiet down a unit? This law pretty much left the decision up to the doctor and the treatment team. As we know from the *Hartford Courant* articles, seclusion and restraint decisions aren't always made with careful consideration, and they can be carried out in punitive and dangerous ways even when they are intended to help. This is why federal law now mandates that every state have a protection and advocacy organization to monitor the use of seclusion and restraint and to investigate allegations of abuse.

Law professor and mental health advocate Elyn Saks pointed out in her memoir, *The Center Cannot Hold*, that at one time restraints themselves were believed to be therapeutic. When she spoke about her own psychiatric hospitalization, the pain, decades after that hospitalization, remained evident in her voice. She recalled the agony of being held in restraints for hours and the indignity of treatment. "My chart," Saks told me, "said to 'restrain liberally.'"

More distressing stories were reported in 1999, when the Centers for Medicare and Medicaid Services published an interim final rule in the Federal Register setting standards to minimize the use of seclusion and restraint. The change was opened to public comment, and CMS received anecdotes from all over the United States. The stories people told were horrifying.

> [The report included] accounts of patients being choked during take-downs even though staff had been trained in proper procedures, and patients suffering broken limbs or other injuries. Other commenters described situations where patients had been placed in restraints for extended periods of time (up to 10 consecutive hours) and staff did not take vital signs regularly, did not offer food, fluids, or use of the toilet at all, or offered them only once while the patient was restrained. Comments also related concerns about the overuse and inappropriate use of restraint or seclusion. One commenter stated that a lawsuit was filed on behalf of a patient dually diagnosed with mental retardation and organic brain syndrome who was placed in restraints 48 times within a six month period. The commenter stated that in the six months after the lawsuit was settled, the patient had only been restrained twice.

In all, CMS got 4,200 comments. Many of those opposed to the rule changes complained that the new policy was a "knee-jerk" reaction to a small number of high-profile events. Some specifically criticized the *Hartford Courant* articles and dismissed the relevance of 142 deaths. Some complained that the new rules would require too much time from staff and that hospitals without a restraint problem were being punished for the negligence of a few.

Dr. Ray DePaulo, chair of the Department of Psychiatry at Johns Hopkins Hospital, talked about his experience leading efforts to reduce the use of restraints.

"Seclusion and restraint have been reduced dramatically, but the result is that on two of our four units we have uniformed security 24/7. We need it because staff and patients were getting assaulted. It has changed the tenor of the units. We're controlling the assaults to a great extent, but to do that, we've got to have a cop walking the beat. I think that's bad; it's degrading the experience of being in the hospital."

The final version of the CMS rules included several reforms: restraints or seclusion could be used only as a last resort and in the least restrictive manner possible to protect the patient or others from harm; restraint or seclusion must be removed or ended at the earliest possible time; and anyone placed in restraints had to be evaluated within one hour by a licensed mental health professional. The new rules also required mandatory training in the application of restraints, as well as a requirement to report deaths related to their use.

The Centers for Medicare and Medicaid Services are responsible for monitoring the quality of patient care in psychiatric facilities. In April 2014, for the first time, CMS published data gathered from 1,753 psychiatric hospitals nationwide so that prospective patients and the general public could see how often seclusion and restraints were used in various states. This information was surprising.

One might have expected that states with a high percentage of patients who are committed—legally found to be both mentally ill and dangerous—would have the most hours of seclusion and restraint use, but in fact there was no significant correlation at all. There was actually a trend toward *less* seclusion and restraint in systems with a high percentage of involuntary patients.

Shouldn't there be some relationship between the clinical status of the patient and the use of restraints? There haven't been enough studies about this to draw any firm conclusions, but some research suggests that non-patient factors—staff perception of a unit's safety, or how well organized and structured the team is—may have more influence than a patient's behavior or dangerousness. If the staff feels supported and safe, they may be less likely to use restraints on patients.

There is also geographic variation in the use of restraints. One study of VA medical centers showed that the use of restraints and seclusion in the Mid-Atlantic and Pacific Northwest regions was substantially lower than in other parts of the United States.

It's hard to understand why some facilities use restraints liberally while other facilities hardly use them at all, particularly when the only data we have are about systems or states rather than individual hospitals. And some hospitals may reduce restraint use merely by transferring dangerous patients elsewhere.

Forensic psychiatrist Paul Appelbaum noted:

In many of the sites that brag that they've eliminated seclusion and restraint, they've been able to do it by transferring their problems somewhere else. They tell you, "we can't handle that type of patient," or they have some route out a back door to a state facility. They are [working] with a very selected patient population, and the fact that they're able to eliminate seclusion and restraint doesn't mean that the patients who needed it have suddenly been contained with gentle talk and Muzak in the background. It's a function of simply who their patient population is.

While patients have died due to improper use of restraints, restrictions on restraint use also carry risk. One example of the problems that can occur took place at the maximum security forensic hospital in St. Peter, Minnesota. Following an effort to decrease the use of restraints, staff injuries in the hospital rose nearly 50 percent between 2011 and 2012, most involving assaults by patients. The prohibition against restraints was so extreme that one patient was even allowed to repeatedly batter his head against a concrete wall.

Hospitals, and the psychiatrists who work in them, are struggling to meet the demands of CMS to decrease seclusion and restraints while also protecting patients from each other. Keeping a watchful eye over all of this are the states' disability law centers. The systematic failure to protect patients or patient injuries due to the improper use of restraints can lead a disability law center to file a class action suit against a hospital on behalf of all patients institutionalized there. While a class action suit can improve hospital conditions, it is a drawn-out, expensive, and time-consuming process that pulls a hospital's resources away from patient care. The risk of a civil rights suit, as well as general legal liability, however, motivates hospitals to create innovative solutions to manage violent or potentially aggressive patients.

The Pennsylvania state hospital system was able to dramatically reduce the use of restraints without any increase in staff injuries. The state mandated that all staff receive annual training in crisis management and verbal de-escalation techniques. Staff-patient ratios were increased, and hospitals formed psychiatric emergency response teams, which mediated crises and debriefed both patients and staff afterward. The restraint reduction program required hospitals to notify the patient's family after any use of restraints if the patient gave permission to do so, and restraint orders were limited to one hour in length. Finally, patients were actively engaged in therapeutic programs, such as vocational training, money management, and illness education, with the goal of preparing them for independent life after discharge.

At Maryland's forensic hospital, the Clifton T. Perkins Hospital Center, chief executive officer David Helsel explained in an interview with the *Boston Globe* his intention to eliminate the use of restraints and seclusion within five years.

"Seclusion and restraints can traumatize or re-traumatize patients and they can lead to injuries of patients and staff. There are a number of compelling reasons to not only reduce, but to eliminate, seclusion and restraints. If you can manage the person's anger and violence using appropriate techniques for just long enough for them to calm down, you can often avoid using restraints entirely." So far, his efforts appear to be paying off. The hospital was given an award by the state for reducing inpatient assaults.

Even with a hospital administration determined to reduce restraint use, however, a hospital can be an unpredictable place, and safety is never guaranteed. Sometimes, a patient is so repetitively assaultive, with an illness that is unresponsive to treatment, that there is no other way to keep the other patients and the staff safe.

The patient who assaulted me had assaulted another staff member earlier in the day. Some people might believe that he should have been placed in seclusion or restraints, and stayed that way throughout the morning. Certainly, that would have prevented the attack on me. But what about the afternoon shift? Or the evening shift? Or the next day? There is no guaranteed safe time to come out of restraints, so there will always be an element of risk. Perpetual restraint is neither a kind nor a realistic solution.

Dr. Daniel Fisher of the National Empowerment Center talked about his own experiences with involuntary treatment and elaborated on the dilemma.

> Seclusion, it's solitary confinement, and they lock the door. I think anyone who is going to put anyone in seclusion should experience it. To not know when you're going to get out and be in a state of mind where you feel completely alone to begin with—I was feeling very disconnected being in a hospital away from home, away from family and friends, and on top of it to be put in seclusion! I actually imagined that my soul left my body and

flew out the window to freedom, and then the next thought I had was that if I ever get out of here, I'm going to become a psychiatrist and then nobody will be treated this way. And then I blacked out, and when I came to, I was in my bed.

I really felt for a while like I lost my soul—I think I've gained it back—but I felt like some of the treatment was just barbaric. And it still goes on—seclusion, restraints, forced medicine. And I recognize, having practiced as a psychiatrist in a state hospital and in a general hospital, that there are times we just don't know what else to do.

In the aftermath of my assault, I was asked if I wanted to file criminal charges against my attacker. I didn't, knowing that in all likelihood he was a very sick person. I didn't think prosecution would be fair or right. When I wrote about my experience later, some mental health professionals applauded my decision while others accused me of excusing bad behavior. Assaultive patients risk seclusion and restraint, but they also risk criminal prosecution and an even worse loss of liberty in a jail or prison. Physical intervention—in rare and limited circumstances—may be the best of the poor alternatives.

D r. Green, the psychiatrist who treated Eleanor, explained that the staff at his hospital make every effort to avoid giving intramuscular medications, but there are times when they do restrain patients and inject them with medications they don't want.

"To give emergency medications, the patient has to be threatening." He noted that behaviors such as pulling the fire alarm, blocking the door to the unit, or entering other patients' rooms—all things that Eleanor did—would be considered reasons for the emergency administration of medications.

In 1989 the California Court of Appeals in *Riese v. St. Mary's Hospital and Medical Center* determined that for a patient to be medicated against his or her will in non-emergency situations, the patient must be found incompetent. Dr. Green talked about the "Riese hearing," as it's now called, which determines if a patient can be involuntarily medicated in non-emergency situations. He noted that the hearing is sometimes held at the same time as the commitment hearing, and this may have been the case for Eleanor, since she only remembers attending one hearing. Her chart indicates that the Riese hearing occurred, and so Eleanor could be required to take medications, even if there were no emergency. Presumably this means that even if Eleanor was calm and reasonable, if she refused oral medications, she could be held down and forcibly injected.

As the days went by, Eleanor improved and started accepting medications by mouth. She explained why she stopped resisting:

What made them stop injecting me? In part, they finally threatened me enough and hurt and mistreated me enough that I was more willing to take the oral medications. Plus, there was the positive influence of my husband. While the injections were still ongoing, my husband pleaded with me to take the oral medications because they had explained to him that they would not stop injecting me until I agreed to take the oral medications. I thought the oral medications were identical to the injected medications, which was why I refused oral medications so adamantly, but in reading the chart I can see it is not so. My husband told me I wasn't going to get out of the hospital until I took the oral meds, so he advised me to just take them to get myself released, so I did.

Involuntary medications are not necessarily equated with injections. Patients sometimes refuse medications, have a court hearing, are told by the judge that they have to take medications, and they then swallow the pills because there is a court order. That doesn't mean that it's a voluntary process. Also, patients may agree to take medications by injection because they work faster, so injections are not always involuntary.

Medications can be administered to a patient in an emergency situation without a court order. Often, this occurs in the ED when someone is agitated, threatening, violent, or physically uncontrollable, and the fear is that they will hurt themselves or someone else.

Each state has different laws about the involuntary administration of medications outside of an emergency situation. In Maryland, the legislation has had some interesting repercussions. The following story is a bit involved, and as of this writing, it's still evolving.

Anthony Kelly is not a man who garners sympathy. He's not a man one would expect advocates and judges to rally for, and he's not a man whose desires one might expect to guide public policy. Kelly has done things that make it easy to despise him.

In March 2002 in Silver Spring, Maryland, a well-to-do suburb of Washington, DC, Kelly assaulted and raped a 60-year-old woman as she walked to her car. He broke her wrist, dislocated her shoulder, pistol-whipped her, and left her face so bloody that she was initially unrecognizable to her own daughter. But she lived. In June of that same year, Kelly stole a car and forced a 20-year-old woman in nearby Wheaton, Maryland, to get into the car with him. He drove to a wooded area and raped her, and like his previous victim, she lived.

Kelly's next known victims were not so lucky. He broke into a single-family, brick colonial home in Silver Spring. He was wearing a wig and a long, fake beard, and he entered the home by breaking through a kitchen window. Once inside, he made his way to a bedroom where he found Erika Smith, a 9-year-old girl. Erika was a shy child with long dark hair. She was beautiful and, despite being shy, was quite popular with her girlfriends. Erika played piano, loved her cats, loved to read, and attended a prestigious private school. On that particular June evening in 2002, she was spending the night with her father so he could take her to the orthodontist the next morning.

Erika was absolutely terrified when she saw Kelly, and she did what every little girl would do: she screamed for her father. Kelly struck the child with his pistol, then shot her in the back of the head. Greg Russell, an accountant, was on the phone with a friend when he heard his daughter scream. He ran to help Erika, and Kelly shot him six times, then fled the house with only a Bible and three dollars. Russell managed to dial 911, but neither father nor daughter survived Kelly's violent home invasion.

Anthony Kelly was also accused of killing a tourist in a Metro station in Washington, DC, three nights later. The evidence linking him to the cases was overwhelming: he had kept possessions from his victims, and his wigs were found in the wheel well of a car he stole and in his home.

While it's every parent's worst fear, the murder of a child by a stranger is a rare event. In 2002, Erika Smith was one of only 11 girls between the ages of 6 and 11 to be killed by a stranger in the United States.

At the time of his violent crime spree, Kelly was on parole; he had been released after an assault charge. He'd had prior convictions for 12 felonies and 24 burglary charges. He was captured by authorities when he ran from a stolen vehicle that was linked to one of the rapes. After his arrest, there were questions about Kelly's mental state and his competence to understand the proceedings against him and to assist with his own defense. In July 2003, he attempted to dismiss his public defenders, stating he didn't trust them. He said his lawyers had a conspiracy against him. This prompted Judge Durke G. Thompson, during a competency hearing, to order Kelly to be moved for a formal evaluation. In September 2003, Kelly was placed in the Clifton T. Perkins Hospital, a maximum security forensic hospital where patients are evaluated and treated for psychiatric disorders.

Admission to Perkins is contingent on an act of violence or alleged violence. Most patients are committed for evaluation prior to a criminal trial, or for treatment after they've been found not criminally responsible (legally insane) for crimes they've committed because of their mental illness. Civilly committed patients who are not criminal defendants may be transferred to Perkins, but only if their behavior is too dangerous to be managed in a less secure state hospital. Prisoners in the state's Division of Correction may be transferred there if they require an involuntary medication panel. On rare occasions, a mentally ill person may be transferred to Perkins directly from an emergency room if he or she is brought in immediately after a serious or bizarre crime and obviously needs inpatient care.

Because most people with mental illness don't commit crimes, or commit only minor, nonviolent offenses like shoplifting or disturbing the peace, forensic hospitals are reserved for the sickest and most high-risk patients. While it may be hard to imagine that anyone would willingly go to a hospital filled with potentially violent patients, some insanity acquittees (people charged with a crime who are found legally insane) in the community do sign in voluntarily when they need hospitalization. Given that an insanity acquittee could be hospitalized for years before earning release, it's understandable that a forensic hospital may become a place where a patient feels comfortable, partly because the staff are familiar.

At Perkins, Kelly was a model patient who never required restraints, seclusion, or any special observation. Because he was delusional and unable to understand the gravity of the charges against him, he was deemed incompetent to stand trial by two psychiatrists. The report they produced was the longest pretrial report ever submitted on a Perkins patient at the time.

When a judge adjudicates criminal defendants to be incompetent to stand trial, they are committed to a hospital for treatment and restoration. Most incompetent defendants are restored within a matter of months, so they can then be tried for their crimes. Some defendants have mental illnesses so severe that they can never be restored to competence. Every state has a statutory time limit beyond which a patient is considered unrestorable, which is generally a year. Maryland is unique because the statutory limit may be as long as 10 years, depending on the crime. Because it's unconstitutional to hold a defendant indefinitely without a trial, once a defendant is adjudicated unrestorable, the criminal charge must be dropped and the defendant freed if he or she doesn't meet the civil commitment criterion of dangerousness due to mental illness.

Of course, all of this assumes that the hospital is actually able to provide treatment. Medication is a major component of treatment for a delusional patient, but because Kelly refused medication while behaving well in the hospital, he remained incompetent to stand trial as a result of his delusional state. This meant that once the statutory time limit ran out, if he were still incompetent but not civilly committable, the hospital would have been required to free him! Clearly, there was a lot at stake in this case, and everyone was concerned.

Kelly asserted that he was innocent, and he did not believe he had a mental illness. While he initially agreed to take medications, he later refused. A clinical review panel heard his case and decided that Kelly could be medicated against his will for up to 90 days. Kelly challenged the finding, and an administrative law judge, Georgia Brady, heard the case.

Dr. Robert Wisner-Carlson was Kelly's treating psychiatrist at Perkins. Wisner-Carlson is an earnest, soft-spoken man from the Midwest with a gentle manner, shaggy hair, a beard, and warm eyes. He is a thoughtful and intelligent man who trained in psychiatry at Johns Hopkins and at the Maudsley Hospital in London. A choir boy in his youth, Wisner-Carlson has a wide variety of interests, including a love of music, with particular interest in the viola, and he has a brown belt in karate.

At Kelly's clinical review panel, Wisner-Carlson testified about Kelly's delusional state:

> He believed that he could represent himself in the cases against him, which were serious cases, and according to his attorney, were charges that wouldn't be dropped and that could result in the death penalty for him. And he wished to represent himself and put himself forward to the case as a pro se litigant, saying that he felt that there is a conspiracy; that his lawyer was part of the conspiracy; that she had lied to him on a number of occasions; and that she had lied to him in particular about a so-called secret search warrant; that she had gotten it inappropriately from the State's Attorney; that she had supposedly told him about a plea bargain that would cap the sentence for all the charges to six years.

Kelly testified that he was not mentally ill, that he was 100 percent certain he was competent to stand trial, and that he did not like taking medication. He didn't find it helpful, and one evening he had the shakes and sweated, circumstances he attributed to the medication. Judge Brady upheld the decision of the clinical review panel:

> I find that Dr. Wisner-Carlson's diagnosis of delusional disorder is, in fact, a reasonable, supportable diagnosis. Next, I have to determine whether the medication prescribed by Dr. Wisner-Carlson has been prescribed for the purpose of treating delusional disorder. Dr. Wisner-Carlson has credibly testified that the medical authorities support treatment of delusional disorder through medication. He has also testified that other psychiatrists in this hospital believe that it is—delusional disorder is treatable through these medications. Therefore, I find that his testimony, that the medication was prescribed for the purpose of treating a mental disorder, to be supported by the evidence. The evidence is also undisputed that Mr. Kelly has refused the psychiatric medications that are listed in the Clinical Review Panel's decision. . . . I do not believe that the side effects are so severe as to make it an unreasonable exercise of professional judgement to administer these medications to Mr. Kelly. Moreover, Dr. Wisner-Carlson has testified that some of Mr. Kelly's symptoms appear to be dissolving after treatment [with] this medication further supporting my conclusion that the administration of medication represents a reasonable exercise of professional judgement.

But Anthony Kelly remained adamant that he didn't want to take psychotropic medications, and he appealed to the Office of Administrative Hearings. The OAH found in favor of the hospital, and Kelly appealed the case to the Circuit Court of Baltimore City.

The circuit court judge relied on an old, overturned state case to decide in favor of Kelly that "for purposes of forcible administration of medication, § 10-708 (g) of the Health—General Article *requires evidence that an involuntarily committed individual is a danger to himself or others in the context of his confinement within the facility in which he has been committed, rather than to society upon release*" (emphasis added).

In other words, no matter how ill a patient was and how dangerous to society at large, he could not be forced to take medications in the hospital *unless he was dangerous while he was inside the hospital*. What a predicament—Kelly could remain delusional, incompetent, and hospitalized for a long time, then be deemed unrestorable and released from the hospital, despite the fact that he was accused of killing several people.

An appeal was filed by the Maryland Department of Health and Mental Hygiene. Because the question was so important, the Maryland Court of Appeals, the state's highest court, agreed to bypass the intermediate appellate court and hear the case directly from the circuit court. Many organizations with an interest in the outcome filed briefs both for and against the decision to medicate Kelly, including the Public Justice Center, the Maryland Disability Law Center, Johns Hopkins Hospital, the Bazelon Center, the ACLU, the National Mental Health Association, the National Council for Community Behavioral Healthcare, and the Maryland Psychiatric Society.

The Court of Appeals of Maryland concluded:

> In a nutshell, the Court proposes to hold that, whenever the psychiatrists in a State hospital to which a criminal defendant has been committed by a court pursuant to § 3-106 of the Criminal Procedure Article (CP) believe it necessary to forcibly medicate the person, the focus must always be on whether, without the medication, the person will be dangerous to self or others within the institutional setting. In the Court's view, whether, without the medication the person will have to remain hospitalized for a significantly longer period than would otherwise be necessary because he or she will continue to be a danger to self or others upon release to the community is, as a matter of law, irrelevant.

So Anthony Kelly could be dangerous, lethally so, and mentally ill, but because he had shown no evidence of being dangerous within the confines of the structured hospital setting, he could not be medicated against his will. How could a court come to a decision like this? How could a panel of judges declare that a known risk to public safety was irrelevant?

In this case, the judges were required to decide what the legislators meant when the clinical review panel law was adopted. The law allowed for involuntary medication if, without treatment, the patient would remain mentally ill with symptoms that caused him or her to be a danger to self or others. The problem was that the legislators didn't clarify the conditions under which the dangerousness should be assessed, and the Kelly case neatly exemplified the dilemma. If the circumstances leading to admission could be considered as evidence of dangerousness, there was no problem—an allegation of multiple murders surely would have met the standard. Opponents of this interpretation were unhappy with it because you can't change the past; a logical conclusion would be that criminal defendants could be medicated at any time, even more than a year after the alleged crime, even if they were behaving appropriately. The other interpretation of dangerousness was the possibility of dangerousness "if released," in other words, if not kept in the contained and structured environment of a secure forensic unit. Opponents of this interpretation disliked it because they felt it required psychiatrists to predict future dangerousness—something the profession has not been particularly good at. The Maryland Court of Appeals had decided it was time to settle the question.

In 2008, after six years of hospitalization, Anthony Kelly was finally declared competent to stand trial for two counts of rape and two counts of first degree murder. He had not taken medication, and it's not clear what exactly had changed in the intervening time, at least not from the public records of the case.

He defended himself and cross-examined his rape victims and the surviving family members of his murder victims. Upon being found guilty of first degree murder, he was sentenced to four life sentences plus an extra 100 years, with no possibility of parole. At his sentencing, Kelly spoke for 29 minutes and addressed the families of his victims, asserting his innocence and instructing them to go on *The Montel Williams Show* with a psychic to learn the truth.

Kelly's story and the legal battle he waged to remain off medication all played out in the criminal courts. This book is about involuntary treatment in civil cases, however, where those being treated have not committed any crime. We include this case because it has implications that have been felt throughout the psychiatric community in Maryland. In that state, like many others, the involuntary medication process did not differentiate between patients who were criminal defendants and patients who weren't:

the same standard and procedure applied to all, and the Kelly decision affected involuntary treatment for every committed patient. It created an odd catch-22 in which a patient who might take medications and become better within a matter of days—the average length of stay in a civil psychiatric unit in Maryland for a committed patient is approximately 12 days—could no longer be medicated if he or she was not dangerous within the facility. Even if patients were known to be dangerous in the community, a situation could exist in which they couldn't be discharged for fear they might hurt someone, but couldn't be medicated to relieve the symptoms that rendered them dangerous.

Dr. Jeffrey Janofsky, an associate professor of psychiatry at Johns Hopkins Hospital and a former president of the American Academy of Psychiatry and the Law, noted, "This clogs up the system. There were patients being held in state hospital beds who could be treated and released. Patients with delusions are the hardest; they don't see themselves as ill, and they don't see a reason to take medications." Janofsky said that in some situations at Johns Hopkins, where he runs the short-stay unit, if a patient was committed—meaning they were both mentally ill and dangerous—but the clinical review panel decided they were not dangerous within the hospital, they were sometimes released. "We can't confine people without treating them."

Janofsky was not aware of any specific negative consequences of letting such patients leave the hospital, though certainly one can imagine bad outcomes.

Different hospitals have different policies. Dr. Steven R. Daviss, a former chair of psychiatry at the Baltimore Washington Medical Center, agreed these situations were not uncommon during his tenure. "We couldn't release dangerous people into the community, so we were left to try to convince them to take medications. Generally, they eventually did, but it typically added two to four weeks to how long they remained in the hospital."

In the years after the Kelly opinion changed the standard for forced medications, different institutions did not come to a consensus on how this changed the standards of care and what made for best practices.

In the *Journal of the American Academy of Psychiatry and the Law*, Yamilka Rolon and Joshua Jones wrote about the case:

The temporal lens through which dangerousness is viewed has been narrowed, as the court indicated that it is not interested in a person's history of violence before hospitalization or potential for violence once released. The danger, by the Maryland Court of Appeals' standard, must now be imminent and immediate and within the walls of confinement. The court even acknowledged that a probable outcome of this ruling is that individuals will be without effective treatment for longer periods; require longer, perhaps indefinite, periods of hospitalization; and incur a greater financial cost. What appears lost in the balancing of the liberty interests of avoiding unwanted medication is that remaining involuntarily hospitalized and under the yoke of an untreated mental illness is, in and of itself, a great loss of liberty.

In Maryland, the dispute over standards for involuntary treatment came to a head in the state legislature. In 2013, several delegates sponsored a bill that would have simultaneously changed the standards for emergency evaluation, for civil commitment, and for involuntary medication. The intent of the bill was to create a definition of "grave disability" in the law, an idea supported by NAMI, that would make it easier to have a patient committed.

While this change might seem minor, the proposal was controversial. Some psychiatrists were already interpreting the term "danger to self" to include situations in which patients were unable to care for their basic physical or medical needs. Other doctors, particularly emergency room physicians, interpreted the term to mean only overt acts of violence against others or suicide attempts. In spite of meetings and conference calls to resolve the difference, ultimately there was no agreement on compromise language, and the bill died in committee.

In 2014, another attempt was made to liberalize the involuntary treatment laws. This time, separate bills were introduced to change civil commitment criteria and the clinical review panel process used for medication over objection. Once again, the "grave disability" proposal died in committee, and the civil commitment law was left unchanged.

At the Maryland Senate Finance Committee hearings on February 26, 2014, the room was packed, and the testimony went on for hours. The point was made that "Maryland is warehousing patients."

Dr. Steven Sharfstein testified about the difficulties his hospital had in getting authorization from insurance companies to keep dangerous patients if they were not receiving medications. "Private insurance companies say this is not active treatment, so they won't pay for the admission."

Linda Raines, the chief executive officer of the Mental Health Association of Maryland, talked about the theory that psychiatric medications may worsen illness. "We don't know the long-term impact of these medicines; we might be creating a lifetime of disability. We need to think before we force people to take them."

And a patient who had been forcibly medicated said she wanted the legislators to understand what forced medication entails: "There is physical and mental trauma to both the patients and the staff. I was involuntarily committed, and psychology interns would demand I take the medications. I was thrown down on the floor by these three guys. I went limp, and they ripped my clothes off, then they shot me with something. One of the guys had his hand around my neck to restrain me. Then they left me in a pile. If that's treatment, then the truth is that a lot of hospitals are not safe places."

That patient's sentiments echo Eleanor's.

By the end of the 2014 legislative session, the clinical review panel law was revised to address the problem created by the Kelly decision. The new law allows Maryland hospitals to involuntarily medicate patients based on three potential dangerousness scenarios: the symptoms and acts that led to the civil or criminal commitment, dangerousness demonstrated within the hospital, or dangerousness if the patient were to be released from the hospital. The Maryland Disability Law Center announced its intention to challenge and appeal the law even before it passed. A challenge is currently pending in Maryland's highest court.

In the cases of violent criminal defendants such as Anthony Kelly, one might ask why his right to refuse medication outweighs the victims' right to get the closure or justice a trial might afford. Furthermore, treatment in a forensic hospital is much more expensive than incarceration in a prison, and taxpayers supported Kelly at a cost exceeding $200,000 per year while he refused treatment. The US Constitution requires that even an unsympathetic defendant like Kelly has a right to be mentally fit for trial, and this right cannot be trumped by any potential impact on the victim or the victim's family.

Fortunately, these serious cases are rare. In most cases, mentally ill defendants are held for misdemeanor crimes, and a refusal to take medication can leave defendants in a facility, waiting to be declared competent to stand trial, sometimes for much longer than the sentence they would have served if convicted.

In situations where there are no criminal issues and a patient is held involuntarily in a psychiatric facility on a civil commitment, we wonder if a somewhat prolonged stay without involuntary medication is necessarily a bad thing, especially if it leaves the patient with a remnant of autonomy and dignity, or at least with a sense that he or she is physically safe while in the hospital. But it's hard to hear the stories of Eleanor and the woman who testified before the finance committee; the methods sound barbaric. It is difficult to imagine that there wouldn't be other options except for the most violent and aggressive of patients.

We don't know what would have happened if Eleanor had not been forcibly medicated; she might have ended up spending more time in the seclusion room she hated so much, or she might have decided sooner to take oral medications on her own in the hope of being released from the hospital. We do assume that her stay might have been longer, but we don't know by how much, and we also assume that the entire experience might have been less physically traumatic. On the other hand, we don't know what would have happened if Eleanor had never been admitted at all.

A patient in a psychiatric unit who refuses medication is not completely without treatment. There are educational groups, occupational therapy, and perhaps individual and group psychotherapy. The rest, support, and freedom from the stresses of everyday life may also have therapeutic benefit. Peer support and a therapeutic milieu can be invaluable. The extra time on the unit may allow for a more accurate diagnosis, especially when the patient can be observed unmedicated. With time to form an alliance with the staff, to watch the successful treatment of other patients, and to have discussions, a patient's fears may be allayed without the trauma of the physical assaults that forcing medications may include. It is most certainly less traumatic if medications are taken "voluntarily," even if begrudgingly. As a society, however, we have become victim to the demands of insurers, who often require justification for every day (if not every hour) of hospitalization, and hospitals in turn encourage, reward, and publicize their ever-shrinking lengths of stay. By this standard, keeping a patient in a hospital for days or weeks longer than would be necessary if they could simply be forced to take medications is unacceptable. But the cheapest care is not usually the best care, especially in the treatment of chronic illnesses where traumatizing patients and turning them away from treatment may ultimately cost society so much more because of the emotional toll these methods take.

We used Maryland as an example in this chapter, but these issues play out in other states as well. Earlier, we discussed the civil liberties of a patient in Vermont. The upshot of the 2014 legislative hearings there was that the state's procedures, including those regarding involuntary medications, were revised. The Vermont Psychiatric Association president, Dr. Margaret Bolton, explained, "The legislature passed a bill that will allow expedited hearings, including commitment and medication hearings simultaneously in cases of extreme dangerousness. They also ordered the creation of an ombudsman to oversee the changes and require that within 24 hours of the initial application by a screener and doctor, a psychiatrist will see the patient and either certify the continued hold or release the patient."

Legal Aid attorney Jack McCullough was skeptical of the Vermont legislation: "I don't agree that it will be limited to cases of extreme dangerousness, and I believe it will, as it was designed to do, result in a further increase in the applications for and use of involuntary medication."

We don't know the ideal time to force medications, nor do we know that they will always be effective. Certainly, patients who are not actively violent should not be forcibly medicated immediately, and having an option to force medicines quickly increases the chance that a patient will be traumatized, while decreasing the motivation of the staff to take the time needed to work with patients in an empathic way. At the same time, leaving patients confined to hospitals for protracted periods—in Anthony Kelly's case, for six years—is not reasonable either. The 2014 legislation in Maryland provides clarification regarding the circumstances that allow for involuntary medication, but will be unlikely to provide definitive answers for all cases.

14 Jim and Involuntary Electroconvulsive Therapy

Eleanor and Lily are bright, articulate people who can tell their own stories easily. Jim (not his real name) was not as fortunate, and most of his story was told to me by his sister Ella (also not her real name) and his psychiatrist, Dr. Adam Rosenblatt, the director of geriatric psychiatry at the Medical College of Virginia (MCV) at Virginia Commonwealth University. At the time of our conversations, Jim was in his sixties, and his story, of late, had been tragic.

When I met him, Jim lived in a nursing wing in a Veterans Administration facility. He was bedridden and quite sad about this. While he did not know what year it was, or even what he was watching on television, he did know that he would not walk again. He was not shy about saying he wanted to go home to his own house, which had been vacant for the previous two years, and to his dog.

Jim grew up on a farm in rural Virginia. His family struggled financially, and Ella said she'd go to bed as a child and pray that her parents could pay the bills so they wouldn't lose the farm.

"We had a hard life growing up, and as the oldest boy, my brother worked really hard."

Ella noted that Jim was the smartest of the children and was always a good student, but with the family's financial stresses, college was out of the question. Jim enrolled in the navy and was stationed on a ship. Jim also told me he'd been on a ship during the Vietnam War, but he couldn't recall where it had been stationed; Ella thought perhaps the South Sea.

During his time in the military, Jim became quite ill. He was hospitalized for months at a time and then discharged from the military on full disability. Ella believed that his diagnosis then was either schizophrenia or manic depressive disorder, and she recalled that he returned home on medication and was jittery and nervous.

Jim was later put on lithium, and despite a few relapses, he did well. He bought his own home; he liked cars and owned two of them. He lived near Ella and saw her often, and he had some friends in town. And he loved his dog. There were ups and downs, but Jim had interests and relationships and things that give meaning to a person's existence.

After 40 years, the lithium damaged Jim's kidneys, and he could no longer take it. He was started on another medication, Haldol, which was given by injection every 28 days. This medication is given by injection because it works slowly over time; it has been found to prevent relapses of psychosis. While it is often used for people who forget to take oral medications, Jim was receiving this medication voluntarily. Unfortunately, he had terrible side effects from the new medicine.

"He was a mess. He walked like he had Parkinson's disease. I sometimes wonder if he wouldn't be better off taking lithium and having dialysis," Ella said.

Jim was having trouble walking, and one day he couldn't get out of the bathtub. He ended up in the hospital and was placed on a psychiatric unit for three weeks. Ella reported, "They kept him in a wheelchair because he was at risk for falling, and then he got a blood clot."

Jim was transferred to a medical floor where he was tied down to keep him in bed so he wouldn't get up and fall. At one point, when he didn't answer the phone, Ella went to the hospital and found him in a coma. "They put him in the ICU, and he was there for 13 days. He nearly died; it was awful," she said.

From there, Jim went to rehab, but Ella said he wouldn't participate with the staff and so they stopped trying. At times he'd get sick (either mentally or physically), and he was sent to five different hospitals. Eventually, he came under the care of Rosenblatt.

"Dr. Rosenblatt was one of the few people who took an interest in my brother," Ella said. "He took him to MCV for ECT [electroconvulsive therapy] when no one could manage him. He'd fuss and he'd fuss, but Dr. Rosenblatt has been wonderful for him."

Rosenblatt reviewed some of Jim's history with me, detailing what had happened before he met Jim.

"As is common in older folks with bipolar disorder, his episodes of mania got closer together and harder to treat, until he was essentially never well anymore. His health also began to fail, probably in part because he wasn't getting effective treatment for his other conditions, like hypertension, because he was so sick with his psychiatric illness. This likely led to a vascular dementia."

Jim had a period of catatonic depression that lasted for weeks. During that time, he remained in bed and was not responsive to others. A feeding tube was placed; he developed bedsores; and, from the lack of movement, he developed severe contractures that left him permanently unable to walk. "A correct diagnosis and involuntary ECT might have spared him all these terrible complications," Rosenblatt said.

In addition, Jim suffered from manias, and at times it was difficult for facilities to manage him. Rosenblatt noted, "When I first met him, he was boisterous, hyperreligious, irritable, not sleeping, and throwing full urinals at the staff. I arranged for his transfer to MCV, where he was given his first course of involuntary ECT."

Modern-day electroconvulsive therapy does not look like the scene in *One Flew over the Cuckoo's Nest* where Randle Patrick McMurphy, the character played by Jack Nicholson, is escorted into a room with shackles on his hands. He lies on the gurney and is instructed to spit out his gum. Conducting gel is placed on his temples and a mouthguard is shoved in his mouth, all without explanation. He is given the treatment with little warning while men in white coats hold down his limbs, and he violently seizes.

Today's ECT looks a little different, but it is not completely different. The patient still lies on a gurney, and professionals in white coats still scurry around the room and do several things simultaneously. The big change is that the patient's vital signs and brain activity are monitored, general anesthesia is given so neither the stimulation nor the seizure is experienced by the patient, and it is not so disturbing to watch. The vast majority of ECT is done as a voluntary procedure, and the patients come willingly, without shackles, threats, or intimidation. It's not a fun procedure, and there are risks and side effects, but it doesn't look like a scene from a horror movie. Patients tolerate it because they are desperate for relief from their psychological pain. ECT is sometimes thought of as a therapeutic relic of an older age, like frontal lobotomies, and some people are surprised to learn that it is still being used.

The ECT suite at Virginia Commonwealth University's Medical Center was filled with computers and medical equipment. Each patient walked in and lay down on a stretcher. An anesthesiologist and a nurse-anesthetist introduced themselves, then inserted an intravenous line and hooked up a heart monitor. A pulse oximeter, a device resembling a clothespin, was attached to the patient's finger in order to monitor blood oxygen levels. The psychiatry resident placed gel and electrodes on the patient's temples or the front of the forehead, where the electric current would be administered. A fast-acting barbiturate put the patient to sleep, and a paralytic agent prevented movement and accidental injury during the seizure.

ECT is typically thought of as a last resort for depression, when symptoms are severe and all other treatment has failed. Because response rates are high and relief may be quick—with symptoms starting to lift within two weeks—it's the treatment of choice for life-threatening conditions such as catatonia. ECT is almost never the first treatment that's tried; it is reserved for situations where the psychopathology is severe and medications either don't work or are not safe to use.

While ECT is one of the most effective treatments offered by psychiatrists today, it also remains the most controversial. The treatment was initially overused after its discovery in the 1930s before any psychiatric medications were available, and it is not benign. Death occurs in approximately one in 10,000 patients. The risk of death is from the risk of general anesthesia, and ECT puts stress on the heart. The most common side effects from the treatment are headaches and memory loss. The headaches can often be managed with medications but still may be severe. The memory loss is often confined to the hours or days surrounding the treatments, but in some instances it can be more pervasive and terribly distressing. These are risks people only take when the condition that needs treatment is absolutely intolerable.

About 100,000 patients a year receive ECT. While it is highly effective for treating depression, it usually requires 8–12 treatments or more for a good response. The relapse rate is also quite high, and patients usually take antidepressant medications after the treatments. Patients who have required multiple courses of ECT and relapsed may elect to undergo maintenance treatments in which ECT is given on a regular basis as an outpatient, usually once a month, even when the patient is having no psychiatric symptoms.

Patients have a variety of reactions to ECT. In the course of asking people about their experiences, we received the following response:

> Ten years ago, I'd just completed my PhD and was about to start a research career. Six years ago, I was desperately depressed and suicidal. Since then, I've had about 100 ECT treatments; the most recent course [was] about 25. ECT has saved my life but cost me myself, and I often struggle with the loss of who I thought I was. I thought I was an intellectual, an award-winning scientist, a researcher. Over the last six years, the treatments—or perhaps the illness?—have cost me my cognitive skills to the point that my boss pulled me into his office and told me he couldn't pay me a researcher's rate any longer because "you just can't think the way I need you to think anymore." That was devastating.
>
> I have lost so many memories that I often am unaware that I haven't remembered something significant that everyone else in the family thinks I should. My research career is over—I can only recall the outline of my PhD research. I have difficulty laying down new memories; my kids are used to me saying, "Sorry, you know mum has a stuffed-up memory." Would I have ECT again? Reluctantly, yes. The last time I had a significant breakdown my kids were present, and their devastation at the prospect that they might never see me again was the only thing that stopped me from acting on my desire to die.

Another woman wrote: "I have had three series of ECT. The third one included maintenance treatments for a period of 18 months (every other week, then every three weeks, and finally every four weeks for several months). I would do it again. My memory losses were small, and when reminded I usually could recall most of them. I have more memory loss from my extended period of major depression than from ECT."

ECT delivers an electric current to the brain, which induces a generalized seizure designed to last 30 seconds to 3 minutes. The seizure is necessary for the treatment to be effective, but no one knows exactly why. Many years ago, one of my psychiatry professors explained it this way: "You know how when the TV doesn't work and you kick it and then it works?" Presumably, the seizure induces a surge of neurotransmitters, but the precise reason for its efficacy remains unknown. There is growing evidence that the seizure triggers similar brain changes as other antidepressant modalities, albeit more robustly and quickly.

The more risky a treatment, the more objectionable it is to force another person to undergo it. Involuntary ECT is given rarely in many places, and it is generally used with very ill, incapacitated patients who are deemed "involuntary" patients because they cannot give consent. In general, they are too psychiatrically ill to communicate in a meaningful way, if at all.

"It's surprisingly easy to do involuntary ECT in Virginia. It's no different than giving involuntary medications," Rosenblatt noted. The judicial process in Virginia entails a hearing with a magistrate, who comes to the hospital, and the patient is provided with an attorney. In addition, there is an independent review of the case by an outside psychiatrist.

As with most procedures for involuntary treatment, the laws vary by state. Dr. Irving Reti is the editor of *Brain Stimulation: Methodologies and Interventions*, a book published in 2015. He heads the brain stimulation unit at Johns Hopkins Hospital in Maryland, where 150–200 patients a year are treated with ECT. Reti estimated that 3 or 4 patients a year are treated with ECT involuntarily. As in Virginia, a court hearing is required, but this entails something different from the routine commitment hearings. These patients, Reti noted, are too ill, often catatonic or psychotic, to verbally refuse or agree. In these instances, the family is in favor of proceeding with the treatment, and the patient lacks the capacity to consent to voluntary treatment.

Reti noted that ECT has been given in the ICU in an attempt to stop ongoing seizures (status epilepticus). When ECT is used to treat a neurologic condition, a court proceeding is not required when the patient can't consent.

Dr. Ananda Pandurangi is the director of brain stimulation therapies at VCU, where Jim was treated. He has worked there since 1984. Pandurangi went to medical school and studied psychiatry in India. When he moved to the United States, he had to repeat his psychiatric training and did so at Syracuse University and Columbia University.

"I chose Syracuse for residency. In India, I had read a lot of American psychiatry, and I wanted to meet Thomas Szasz. He didn't believe that schizophrenia existed and was very much opposed [to] involuntary treatment. At the psychiatry clinics in Bangalore, the patients would line up a hundred deep. At the end of the day, we'd send . . . away [those we hadn't seen] and tell them to come back tomorrow. I didn't understand this idea of forced care, and I wanted to talk to him."

Pandurangi directs ECT treatment at MCV, and he examines every patient who is referred for treatment; the decision to proceed is ultimately his, and he has seen a tremendous number of patients over the years. Other hospitals, including some that have their own ECT facilities, refer their difficult cases to him. He estimated that MCV treats 110 patients a year with ECT and that 15–20 of these patients are involuntary. Many are involuntary because they lack the capacity to give consent, but some patients do say they don't want the procedure.

"I have three reasons to treat with involuntary ECT: catatonia, bipolar mania that hasn't responded to medication, and severe depression with psychosis. With catatonia, medications can make the condition worse or cause serious complications."

Pandurangi talked more about what it means to be an involuntary patient:

When it is clear that a person comprehends what is being offered as treatment and understands the basic elements of it, and verbally declines, the situation is clear enough: ECT, if implemented, would be "involuntary." To my knowledge, we have never performed this type of involuntary ECT. Similarly, even when a patient has exhibited serious suicidal behavior, but understands and declines ECT, I don't feel we should implement it against their wishes. In my mind, this is a genuine choice he or she is making. However, in reality, the picture is never black or white.

Thus, we might have someone who becomes catatonic—mute, staring, posturing. His mother brings him to the hospital and expects us to give him ECT, which helps for short periods of time. He neither says yes nor no to ECT. He simply stands in his room or the hallway. We obtain a court order for involuntary ECT. With some cajoling and encouragement, he cooperates with all aspects of the procedure and never physically resists it. We call these situations "passive consent." However, this is not sufficient to implement ECT, and so we petition the court and there is a hearing before we proceed. Yet another situation is one where the person is overtly psychotic, and he is verbal and refuses ECT. But his other behaviors indicate psychosis, such as bizarre delusions, frequent hallucinatory behavior, regressed behaviors such as soiling, etc. It is in these cases that the magistrate and court order really make a difference. I have one other rather arguable criterion that I use in determining involuntary ECT. I require the significant other or legal next of kin to assent to ECT. If such a person is opposed to ECT, we will not proceed with it. However, if such person does not wish to get involved, I am kind of stuck. Sometimes, we have chosen to approach the ethics committee to help guide the decision.

Both Rosenblatt and Pandurangi see the procedure as life-saving. They described a patient population that languishes in state hospitals, some of whom—like Jim—require tube feeding for survival or require massive doses of antipsychotics to contain their behavior. Other states, however, manage without involuntary ECT or use it much less often than the Medical College of Virginia does.

"They manage, but what does that mean?" Pandurangi asked. "There are patients who we see who benefit, and in other places those patients remain in a facility with no quality of life. It is wrong to let people suffer when there is a treatment they can be offered to help them. There was one patient I saw in his early fifties, and he hadn't been eating or responding for months. When we gave him ECT, he got better. He'd been at the other hospital for a long time, and when I asked, I learned that their treatment plan was to move him to a hospice facility to die."

Pandurangi talked about another patient he had seen recently. The man was completely mute and was not eating.

"We had to give him treatments in the intensive care unit. After the first treatment, the nurse called me and said he was talking. That's unusual; it usually takes a few treatments. I went to see him, and he thanked me for doing the procedure. He told me, 'You know, I wanted to speak, but I couldn't. I tried. I don't want them to think I didn't try.'"

While every patient does not express such appreciation, neither Rosenblatt nor Pandurangi was aware of any patients who felt traumatized by involuntary ECT. "I won't swear to this," Pandurangi said, "but no one is calling me to complain." They both felt good about the care they were giving and had no question as to whether it was the right thing to do.

"I wish it was pleasant," Pandurangi said. "The waiting area should be more comforting and colorful, and in the recovery area we should have therapy dogs."

Pandurangi does not simply rubber-stamp ECT at VCU. He routinely turns patients away or recommends other therapies. He described one situation in which he was asked to consult on a patient in a state facility. The patient wouldn't eat and wouldn't talk.

"I got there, and he spoke to me. He told me that he wasn't eating until his legal situation had been decided. This was behavioral; it isn't something that we do ECT for. But after that, the facility stopped referring patients to me."

Pandurangi mentioned another case where the patient had made a serious suicide attempt and had been placed on the psychiatric unit, where he was continuing to try to take his own life. The staff felt that time was of the essence and that ECT might alleviate the patient's depression faster than waiting for medications to work. "I told them to wait; he had never been treated with an antidepressant before. I wanted them to try medications for at least a week before even considering ECT."

Dr. Pandurangi's expertise in electroconvulsive therapy makes him the natural person to turn to for consultation in the Richmond area. Since most general psychiatrists don't do ECT, the American Psychiatric Association recommends they seek consultation with someone like Pandurangi even when the patient voluntarily agrees to the treatment. This makes sure that less intrusive treatments have been exhausted and that the patient is competent to make the treatment decision. ECT is the only psychiatric treatment in which the professional standards recommend a higher level of review than is required by law, even for *voluntary* treatment. After all, no second opinion is required to prescribe a medication or to conduct psychotherapy.

This is because the practice of ECT and the legal regulation of it are so controversial. There is a movement among opponents of ECT to have the practice abolished. ECT was first used in the United States in 1938, the same year the federal government gave the Food and Drug Administration the authority to monitor and regulate medical devices. Because ECT machines were already on the market and in use, there was no requirement that they undergo the usual tests for safety and efficacy that new medical devices must have today.

The psychiatric survivors organization MindFreedom International encouraged its members to write letters opposing the classification of ECT machines as safe; the group's preference was to have it classified as a "premarket" experimental device—a classification that would have substantially cut back its use.

An expert panel was assembled to advise the FDA about the issue in 2011. So far, no recommendation has been made, and there have been no new restrictions on the use of ECT.

This is not to say that the practice is entirely unregulated. Although 33 states have no regulations or laws governing the use of ECT, in 5 states civilly committed patients can only be given ECT after a judicial hearing, and the need for the treatment must be proven by clear and convincing evidence.

Eleanor never had ECT, even though her symptoms were initially difficult to control and required high doses of several medications. ECT either was never considered as an option, or it was not mentioned to Eleanor or Frank nor recorded in her medical record. She knows about the treatment from her own research, and she has watched a YouTube video of a woman with schizophrenia discussing her recovery after ECT. It's unlikely that Pandurangi would have considered her a candidate for involuntary ECT, even though it took weeks to control her mania and the high doses of medications were causing side effects. In general, he suggests using ECT for severe mania if there is no reasonable improvement in two weeks, but by that point in her hospital stay, Eleanor had become notably calmer, so again he would not have pursued involuntary ECT for her, even if she had been in his facility in Virginia. I'll also venture a guess that since Eleanor's husband was disturbed by her treatment generally, he would have objected, and for that reason as well involuntary ECT would not have been an option.

"In California ECT can be given to patients without their consent which I find scary and horrible considering the side effects of losing memory," Eleanor wrote. "I consider part of my essence to be my sharp mind and stored memories of loved ones and my life's history. I think when we lose our memories we lose who we are. I *do* think there can be a profit motive on the part of the clinicians which makes it alarming to me that the very same psychiatrist who can declare a psychiatric inpatient too ill to release can order ECT against the patient's will as well."

California's ECT laws are fairly strict, although this information may not have reassured Eleanor. Even voluntary patients who consent to ECT must have their competency and consent reviewed by three physicians. Involuntary patients are given legal counsel and can challenge the treatment in court.

For Jim, the logistics of ECT did not go smoothly. Jim was involuntarily hospitalized on the psychiatric unit at MCV with a commitment order by a judge that lasted for 30 days. Involuntary ECT was also authorized. Partway through his course of ECT, Jim developed a medical complication and was transferred to a general hospital unit for treatment. During that time, his commitment order expired. An independent evaluator needed to authorize a transfer back to a psychiatric unit—the same process that we previously described for all involuntary psychiatric admissions in Virginia.

"The evaluator noted that Jim had improved so much that he no longer met criteria for involuntary admission. He was lucid and said he didn't want more ECT," Rosenblatt said. "They refused to give my patient back despite my protestation that his treatment was incomplete and that he would swiftly relapse!"

Jim did agree to return to the psychiatry unit voluntarily, but he couldn't be convinced to have more ECT. He was discharged back to the VA facility—improved, but not well. He was eating on his own, the feeding tube had been removed, his bedsores had healed, and he was able to get around in a wheelchair. Soon after, however, he became manic again. He was returned to the MCV psychiatry unit as an involuntary patient and was court-ordered to have involuntary ECT. When he became well, he consented to having maintenance ECT treatments on a regular basis. He also signed over a power of attorney to his sister to consent to ECT again, even over his objections. In doing so, he permanently became a voluntary

ECT patient, a concept that is a bit difficult to digest since most people would think that patients should have a right to change their minds, but this was an option that Jim relinquished.

Rosenblatt said, "Despite our previously adversarial relationship, he likes me very much now and is always happy to see me. He socializes and participates in activities."

Jim's story is not one of great success. His psychiatric illness had been so severe that the only way he could manage to live in the community was to take medications, and while they helped him to function for decades, the medications eventually damaged his physical health. His mental illness, however, was intractable; without treatment, he became too ill to be managed even inside a facility.

Shortly after we finished writing this chapter, I received an email from Dr. Rosenblatt:

> I'm sorry to tell you that "Jim" has recently passed away. His sister called me to tell me that he sounded confused on the phone and I called the VA to check on him and learned that he had developed an infection. He had already been transferred to the medical service from his usual long-term care unit. I went to see him the next day and he was out of sorts, but he recognized me and was pleased to see me. Things spiraled down over the next few days as he developed sepsis, hemolytic anemia and multi-organ failure and died. Everyone on the inpatient unit was very sad to hear of his death because we had invested a great deal of energy into his care, and because he was a pleasant and cheerful presence when he would come in for his monthly maintenance treatments. I tried to cheer the staff up by reminding them that he had almost certainly lived for two additional years because of our treatment and that most of that time had been spent in good spirits and interacting socially with his sister, the staff and other veterans, and also that he had been a religious man who was at peace with God when he died.

Involuntary ECT is rare, and the cases we have presented in this chapter are extreme. The Medical College of Virginia is a tertiary care center, a place where other facilities refer their most difficult cases. In other chapters focusing on patients, we have chosen people who were able to articulate how they felt about their treatments, and hearing how bright Jim was, there certainly was a time when he might have given compelling arguments about his treatments, but that was not the case when I saw him. Jim, an impaired person in dire circumstances whose other options were exhausted, vividly illustrates the difficult decisions surrounding this provocative treatment.

Five

INVOLUNTARY OUTPATIENT COMMITMENT

The system is a mess. Our perspective is that liberty must be expanded
for people with mental health problems, through real choices and the
opportunity to get one's needs met without a court order. We also assert
that engagement in quality mental health care is fundamentally important,
particularly for people with the most serious conditions. These perspectives,
seemingly in conflict, can in fact be aligned.

In the mental health system we seek, care would be early and based
on personal preferences, and services would be welcoming to families.
Assisted outpatient treatment would be more widely available and much
less frequently used—because a system offering early and good care in a
collaborative approach would result in less need for extreme measures.

—*Liberty and Recovery: Resolving a Mental Health Dilemma*,
Scattergood Foundation, Spring 2014

15

Lily was discharged from the hospital, and then she moved to another state. She realized that in her tenuous condition, she needed the support of her family while she continued the long process of healing. She went to see a psychiatrist willingly, and from then on, her treatment was voluntary.

Eleanor was discharged to a partial hospitalization program, also known as a day hospital. The patient goes to the hospital for treatment each day—often between the hours of 8 a.m. and 3 p.m.—but returns home for the evenings, weekends, and holidays. Day programs are generally voluntary. Eleanor's perception, however, was that she had to attend, not because of a medical need, but because she had been committed to treatment by a judge. She continued to see Dr. Green at the day program for three weeks after her discharge.

Eleanor finished her treatment in the day hospital in October. She continued outpatient treatment for a few months with a psychiatrist she didn't like and a psychologist who "kept trying to get me to accept my illness." On her own, she began to taper her medications. The following March, she began to see Dr. Charles Johnston at the suggestion of a friend, in part because he had the reputation of using medications as a last resort. With his help, she came off all medications, and she continued to see him for years for psychotherapy, until they mutually agreed that she was better and did not need continued treatment.

For both Lily and Eleanor, outpatient treatment was helpful, and they went voluntarily. But not every patient who is discharged from the hospital goes voluntarily to treatment. For those patients who have been repeatedly committed to the hospital and who either refuse to attend treatment or are unlikely to comply, 45 states have laws that allow magistrates to order patients to get treatment with a mental health professional. There are many terms for these laws: outpatient civil commitment, assisted outpatient treatment (AOT), mandated outpatient treatment, and community treatment orders. Sometimes, outpatient commitment is called by the name of its legislation: Kendra's Law in New York and Laura's Law in California are named for the murdered victims of people who were mentally ill.

The term most commonly used is AOT, but there are those who are quick to say that "assisted outpatient treatment" is a euphemism—it isn't "assisted," it is court-ordered, and the wording deceptively masks the involuntary nature of the treatment. For this reason, we have chosen to use the term "outpatient commitment" as we discuss court-ordered outpatient care.

I had hoped to focus this chapter on a family in which a member had benefited from outpatient commitment. I found such a family in Arizona, but once the mother realized that this book would be a balanced view of the issues, she declined an interview for herself and her adult child. "For me, there is no balance. This is a medical issue, and the need is clear," she said.

I tried to persuade her that allowing me to write about her family would give her views a voice, but she refused unless I could promise that the message of the book would be wholeheartedly in favor of involuntary treatment. Instead, I found another person to tell her story about outpatient commitment.

Marsha's (not her real name) psychiatric history began at the age of 13 with a serious suicide attempt. Her recovery would prove to be long and difficult with bumps in the road as well as some unexpected twists and turns, not the least of which was her ultimate success.

As a young adult, Marsha was in her therapist's office one day and became angry. "I got mad and kicked the door," she recalled. "Unfortunately, it was glass, and it shattered."

From there, Marsha was sent to the state hospital as an involuntary patient because she was deemed to be in a psychiatric crisis. "I told them I would be happy to sign in. I wanted treatment, and I've always been willing to take medications. But they told me the state would only pay for hospitalizations for involuntary care, so even though I wasn't psychotic, I was committed."

Marsha stayed in the state hospital for nine months, not because she was too sick or dangerous to be in the community for that entire time, but because there was nowhere to send her after discharge. Marsha was not alone in this predicament. Committed patients in Delaware were hospitalized for so long while they waited for housing that the US Department of Justice began an investigation of the problem. The investigation lasted for years and culminated in a 2011 mandate for more community-based services.

When Marsha was finally discharged, she left the hospital with a court order that stated she had to continue with psychiatric treatment, despite the fact that she was not protesting the idea that she needed help. Here, too, nothing was unusual. She was told that court-ordered treatment after release was a matter of protocol for patients discharged from the state hospital. Her court-appointed attorney met with her a few minutes before the hearing but did nothing to advocate for her. Her commitment hearing lasted 5–10 minutes. She liked and respected her psychiatrist and was willing to see him for treatment voluntarily, but he told the judge why he thought continued commitment was necessary, and the hearing was over. She was told, "This is the way we do things."

Marsha had never been psychotic. She was diagnosed with major depression and borderline personality disorder. Nevertheless, she stayed on court-ordered treatment for two years and had to attend recommitment hearings every six months. She never had the opportunity to testify.

Marsha's experience seems to have been typical for patients in Delaware. Chris Devaney is the chief operating officer of Connections, an organization that provides behavioral health services to 30,000 clients across Delaware. He confirmed what Marsha said.

"In Delaware, you could get a ham sandwich on outpatient commitment. There was no challenge to commitments, no testimony."

Marsha's story sounds familiar. In chapter 6, we discussed Mrs. E. P. W. Packard, whose husband signed her into the hospital without a hearing or any opportunity to challenge her commitment. We also mentioned Catherine Lake, an elderly woman with dementia who was kept in the hospital even though she was not dangerous to anyone. Those situations happened decades ago, before the civil rights era and before mandatory due process protections were put in place for psychiatric patients. How could

Marsha have been committed to treatment so easily from 1998 to 2000? The answer lies in the interpretation of one short phrase at the heart of Lake's legal challenge. In her case, the court established the requirement to consider the "least restrictive alternative" to hospitalization. For some states, commitment to outpatient care was that alternative.

Outpatient commitment is one of the most controversial aspects of involuntary psychiatric care. Autonomy over medical decisions is highly valued in US society, and, in the name of autonomy, we allow people to make poor decisions that may cost them their lives and may cost taxpayers countless dollars. We allow people to choose to smoke, own guns, and ride motorcycles without wearing helmets. They can refuse treatment for cancer, even a highly treatable cancer with a good prognosis for cure. We allow people with coronary artery disease to smoke, eat ice cream, lead sedentary lifestyles, and refuse to take medication for high cholesterol or have medical follow-up. There is no organization that mandates good judgment or adherence to recommended medical care. In all other fields of medicine, people make their own decisions about their medical treatment unless they are incompetent and do not understand the proposed treatment along with its associated risks and potential benefits.

Those who advocate for laws that allow for court-ordered outpatient psychiatric care contend that mental illness is different: patients don't know they have a disorder, and so they cannot make the informed decision that they would have made when well. Yet people frequently choose not to follow medical advice. Up to half of patients don't take medication—any medication—as prescribed, even without the issue of a mental illness. If people incorrectly decide that the *possibility* of side effects outweighs the potential benefit of taking a medication, or if they simply don't believe in taking pills, we don't issue court orders to make them take their medication, and we don't confiscate their cookies if they have diabetes.

Advocates for involuntary outpatient treatment point to the frequent and sometimes tragic consequences of untreated severe mental illness in order to justify its use. They assert that the coercion of court-ordered community care can mitigate the risk of homelessness, violence, suicide, and repeated cycles of incarceration or hospitalization.

Outpatient treatment orders usually contain requirements to keep appointments and to adhere to medication regimens, but enforcement can be difficult. While most medications are given to outpatients in the form of daily oral tablets or capsules, in psychiatry there is an option to treat psychosis with long-acting injectable forms of antipsychotic medications. For patients who don't comply with treatment, or who simply forget to take their pills, injections offer an easy solution, and they are effective in preventing relapse. The vast majority of these long-acting injectibles are given on a voluntary basis to patients who don't like getting ill or who have trouble with compliance. However, injections are also often given to people who have involuntary treatment orders.

Proponents of outpatient commitment see noncompliance with medication to be a result of anosognosia—a biologically based lack of insight into the fact that an illness is present—but this view understates the possibility that some patients object to the side effects from these treatments. While psychiatric treatments work wonderfully for some people, they don't work for everyone, and they make some people lethargic. Some medications can cause agitation, disabling tremors, sleepiness or sleeplessness, irreversible movement disorders, loss of sex drive, weight gain, kidney and thyroid diseases, and a predisposition to heart disease, stroke, and diabetes. Some people have no side effects and see only positive results, while others do have side effects but decide that medications are worth it to be able to live a functional life without psychic torment. These are difficult decisions, which we would prefer patients make for themselves with the guidance of their doctors.

The issue is even more complicated, however. In the throes of a psychotic illness, patients may incorrectly believe their food is being contaminated or the medication is poison. As Lily pointed out, there is nothing pleasant about these types of delusion. People with paranoid delusions who believe they are being followed, watched, targeted, and persecuted live in a state of torment. While it feels wrong to force someone to take medications, it also feels wrong to leave a tormented and distressed person to suffer needlessly when medicine may well offer relief. The issue is further complicated when the patient has a history of becoming violent and when treatment decreases the risk of future violence.

Marsha did well on outpatient commitment, in large part due to her determination to get better. While she reported that she was never psychotic and never unwilling to get treatment, most of us can understand why her therapist was frightened when Marsha shattered the glass door.

"I really bought into treatment. I had given up believing I would ever get better, but then I had a psychiatrist who told me there was no reason I could not turn things around. It helped me change my attitude."

Marsha also noted that she pursued treatments that were not easily available, specifically dialectical behavioral therapy for borderline personality disorder. When she couldn't access this treatment, she bought a workbook and went through the exercises with the help of her psychiatrist. "It helped me change my thought processes, and I started to have healthier relationships," she said.

In addition, Marsha attended peer support groups for people with psychiatric disorders. She received government disability benefits for many years, but eventually she improved enough to take a part-time job in a retail store.

Even after her outpatient commitment ended, Marsha continued to do well. She finished her college degree and then became a peer counselor for other people with mental health issues. She decided to start a peer support group, so she wrote a grant proposal and got funding. The group was a success.

"I got into cooking, so I'd bring in food to the groups, and people would come in droves," Marsha said.

Marsha was hired by an assertive community treatment team as a peer specialist, and she spent more than two years working with patients, many of whom were on outpatient commitment orders. It was in this capacity that she saw patients being brought into the hospital to get injections. Her perspective on involuntary care has been influenced by what she saw both as a patient and as a provider.

"For some people, they do force them to take medications," Marsha noted. "We saw people all the time with serious side effects. They would have muscle spasms or be drugged out, or they couldn't function, and they'd shuffle around, but they would still be sent to the hospital to get their shots if they missed getting them."

Marsha still worries a little about repercussions from having been on a commitment order. Several years ago, she got into a verbal altercation with another woman in a parking lot. While there was no physical violence, things got heated, and the police were called. Marsha said that the police were immediately able to pull up the fact that she had been a psychiatric patient on an outpatient commitment order, and she felt uncomfortable.

In addition to her work with the ACT team, Marsha has been a part of the Delaware Consumer Recovery Coalition, an advocacy and recovery-oriented group. Marsha is currently completing her studies for an advanced degree in social work, and once again, we're delighted to share a story with a happy ending.

16 Outpatient Commitment on the Books

Outpatient commitment laws have been in existence since the 1980s. The best known of these programs was implemented in New York after Andrew Goldstein, a man with a psychiatric illness, pushed Kendra Webdale to her death on a subway track in 1999. Goldstein suffered from schizophrenia, and a *New York Times* account noted, "His lawyers blamed his failure to take antipsychotic medication for Ms. Webdale's death and said the state mental health system had repeatedly sent him back to the streets despite a history of violent behavior and his own requests for treatment." The New York statute, Kendra's Law, was named for the victim. Although his lawyer blamed medication noncompliance for the crime, a jury rejected this insanity defense, and Goldstein is currently in prison serving 23 years for second degree murder.

New York's implementation of assisted outpatient treatment is unique because it was accompanied by $125 million in funding to the mental health system in fiscal year 2000–2001. In addition, money is allocated annually for the implementation of Kendra's Law. For that same fiscal year of 2000–2001, $32 million was allocated.

New Yorkers placed on outpatient commitment are moved to the top of waiting lists for housing, and they are given case management services or followed by assertive community treatment teams. To be considered for outpatient commitment, patients are required to have two or more hospitalizations in a 36-month period due to noncompliance, or have a history of acts or threats of violence in the previous 48-month period. Outpatient commitment is generally reserved for those who have been repeatedly hospitalized and is used to transition from inpatient care to the community. Since 1999, more than 13,000 petitions have been filed to place patients on outpatient commitment in the state of New York; 97 percent were granted, and just over 65 percent of these have been in New York City.

Dr. Ryan C. Bell is the medical director of the Steve Schwarzkopf Community Mental Health Center in Rochester, New York. A third of Bell's caseload are people on outpatient commitment. His perspective is colored by his professional experiences. Before he became a doctor, Bell was a district attorney in Alaska; after medical school, he did his psychiatric training in Washington state, where the implementation of outpatient civil commitment is much different than it is in New York.

In a typical community mental health center, a full-time psychiatrist carries a caseload of 300–1,000 patients or more. Bell works in a setting where each psychiatrist follows 80 patients. He noted that few of his patients object to being on a court order.

Only in about 5 percent of the cases do the patients say, "I'm so opposed to this that I'm going to go to court and fight it." In 95 percent of the cases, they say, "All right, I'll do it," and they don't challenge it. So what percentage do it because they're fed up and they want to get out of the hospital, but they don't think they need it? It depends. Most people understand that we think this is going to help them, and they'll agree to it, because they see that we genuinely and honestly believe that this is going to help them meet their goals.

Bell talked about the typical patients he sees on outpatient commitment.

The patients have schizophrenia, schizoaffective, or a severe form of bipolar disorder. They've been hospitalized at least five times in their lives; some of them have been in the hospital a dozen or more times. There are so many hospitalizations and uncountable Emergency Department visits, and the majority have a history of violence toward themselves or others. Invariably, they are folks who are extraordinarily psychotic and unable to care for themselves when they are not on medication, and a significant number—I'd say 75 percent of them—have residual symptoms, so that even after we've maximized medication, they still have significant symptoms that make it difficult for them to live independently in the community.

Bell discussed the care that mandated outpatients receive. When someone is court-ordered to treatment, they receive a visit from the social worker who oversees the program in Monroe County.

She tells them, "This is not about forcing you to do something you don't want to do. This is not about us punishing you. This is about us working with you to get the life that you want. You don't want to be in jail, you don't want to be in the hospital, and these are things we can agree on. We may disagree with why you are in the hospital or in jail, or whether you have a mental illness or not, but we can both agree that you don't want to be in jail or the hospital."

Bell went on to explain that the services available to patients on outpatient commitment are different than those available to voluntary patients. "It's a lot harder to access care if you're not on AOT. If you have someone who needs outreach services, there are not many slots. Right now, we're the only ones who will send a doctor or a social worker into the community."

He continued, "We mandate people to services, but if the services aren't any good, then it doesn't help to mandate them. You've got to have the services in the community."

Bell was positive about his work with committed patients in Rochester. So was everyone else I spoke with in New York.

Henry Dlugacz is an attorney in New York City who represented St. Vincent's Hospital at outpatient commitment hearings.

"Where you stand depends on where you sit," he said. In his experience, outpatient commitment was used as a means of transition from the hospital to the community, and patients were often told that if they went along with the AOT order, the hospital would discharge them. A commitment order counterintuitively became a fast track to discharge. "As the hospital's lawyer, I was in the strange position of being hounded by the patient's lawyer saying, 'Can't you get that petition in for court this Tuesday? My client wants to get out.'"

Dlugacz discussed the ideology of Kendra's Law. "At some point, we have to get past all the touchiness and decide what's good public policy, what helps people, and what's a good use of scarce resources. It's easy for me to say—not that people don't have legitimate concerns—but at some point, it becomes this whole polarizing thing that you're 'for' or you're 'against,' and I don't know that that gets us anywhere productive."

Dr. Paul Appelbaum talked about his experience in New York:

> We've got lots of data to suggest that, in general, it's been very positive in that there are lower rates of hospitalization, lower rates of arrest, higher rates of medication use, higher numbers of outpatient visits, and just about any measure you would look at would show that people who are outpatient committed do better than similar people who are not, even people who have pretty good service packages available to them. Almost by definition, you are selecting for a group that is a low-insight group, a group that is more likely to either not recognize that they are ill or not recognize that they need treatment. The problem with a lot of the advocacy for outpatient commitment as led by the Treatment Advocacy Center is that they seem oblivious to this exact issue, to the need to provide additional services if outpatient commitment is actually going to be used and be effective. Their advocacy has focused on getting the statutes passed in one state after another, and they've been successful. In California, the effect has been that there's a statute in place, but there are no new resources to support it, and it rarely gets used.

The National Alliance on Mental Illness, in conjunction with the Treatment Advocacy Center, has been instrumental in getting such laws passed, and interest in outpatient commitment increased after the Newtown school massacre in 2012. Presently, 45 states have outpatient commitment laws, but as Appelbaum and Bell mentioned, there can be a big difference between having a law on the books and actually being able to implement it.

In one national survey, more than half the states with outpatient commitment laws reported that they did not regularly use them. In the states with such laws, it wasn't unusual for the law to be implemented in only a single part of the state. While New York dedicated funding to expand services, Maryland declined to introduce outpatient commitment legislation because of the potential cost. Even in states with established laws, outpatient programs may be reluctant to accept committed patients due to concerns about risk, particularly if the clinic was not involved in creating the treatment plan. In 2005, only 1.7 percent of all of New York's public mental health patients were committed to outpatient care. Finally, a mere lack of familiarity with the law could explain some geographic variation. In one survey of 739 psychiatrists, more than half answered incorrectly when asked if their state allowed for outpatient civil commitment. Another quarter of the respondents admitted they did not know. A review of all the national outpatient commitment laws reveals that there is tremendous variability regarding who is eligible for commitment, how noncompliance is managed, when commitment should be used, and which services are routinely part of involuntary outpatient care.

While most laws don't specify that a patient must have a particular diagnosis, Oklahoma law requires that the patient have schizophrenia, bipolar disorder, or major depression with suicidal intent. Louisiana, North Dakota, and Nebraska allow outpatient commitment only for a substance abuse diagnosis. West Virginia is one of the few states that allows commitment for people with intellectual or developmental disability. Some laws require a history of previous inpatient civil commitments, while others include voluntary admissions. Still other states don't require previous admissions at all, which seems contradictory when one common justification for outpatient commitment is that it is a means of reducing revolving-door admissions. Many state laws require that a patient be either unable or unwilling to consent to voluntary treatment; in other words, the court must find that the patient demonstrated either treatment refusal or a lack of mental capacity to give informed consent. Other states do not require a capacity assessment and may base commitment solely on a *risk* of mental deterioration leading to future dangerousness. If this weren't all confusing enough, in Virginia the patient must *possess* capacity—in other words, he or she must be able to understand and comply with the treatment agreement.

Marsha, whose story was in the previous chapter, was placed on outpatient commitment as part of a discharge plan, a process that is sometimes called a "conditional release" from the hospital. In states other than Delaware, outpatient commitment may be offered at an inpatient commitment hearing as an alternative to hospitalization. It can also be offered as a "preventive" treatment, before the need for admission, for those who are at risk of decompensation in the community but who don't yet meet the criteria for hospitalization. So, depending on where patients live, they may be considered for mandated outpatient treatment prior to inpatient admission, early in the admission process at a commitment hearing, or upon release.

What happens when a patient doesn't follow the outpatient commitment order?

Marsha, in her capacity as a peer counselor on an ACT team, recalled three times when someone was stopped by the police for an unrelated issue and was then arrested when the police discovered that the person had violated his or her treatment order. In these cases, the patients didn't even necessarily know they were on outpatient commitment orders! A homeless patient without an address might never receive a notification to go to court for outpatient commitment proceedings. In Delaware, failure to comply with treatment can land people in jail, even if they've never committed a crime.

Dr. Bell talked about his experiences in Seattle. "Outpatient commitment there had *teeth*!" In Washington, a noncompliant patient on outpatient commitment could be hospitalized for up to six months without any additional hearings or the need to meet specific criteria, but as Bell noted, resources were scarce and beds were difficult to come by. He didn't feel commitment worked when the patient was mandated to treatment in a system that was not able to care for them with more intensive community services or with short-term hospitalizations when they relapsed. Since then, Washington state's bed shortage has been highlighted by the problem of boarding psychiatric patients in the Emergency Department—in other words, holding them for a long time while waiting for an open bed. A state court ruled that this practice was unconstitutional. In 2015, changes were made to the outpatient commitment laws in Washington that have made it more difficult to hospitalize a patient who does not comply with a court order for outpatient care.

Bell noted that the "teeth" in the Washington system contrasted with New York's laws. In New York, patients who missed an outpatient appointment or refused to comply with treatment could be picked up by the police and brought to the emergency room for evaluation. But patients had to be released if they did not meet the standard commitment criteria of being dangerous to themselves or others.

"In New York," Bell said, "the only way to return someone to the hospital is to make a new finding that they are an imminent danger to themselves or others, or are gravely disabled—even if they have just been released early from a 60-day commitment order, stopped outpatient treatment, and are showing significant clinical symptoms. It's a very different legal environment."

In Ohio, where Lily was hospitalized, Dr. John Morcos is a psychiatrist who provides expert testimony for the probate court in Franklin County. Morcos said that about 80 percent of the time, patients are not opposed to outpatient commitment. The orders, he noted, were for 90 days, and patients are often lost to follow-up.

"It requires an extensive treatment plan. It's very labor-intensive, and mental health centers don't have the money or staffing to implement it. The system breaks down, and follow-up is difficult when patients do not comply."

This highlights another problem with outpatient commitment laws. Even when civil commitment criteria or bed space aren't issues, a patient can still simply abscond from treatment. In fact, the gunman responsible for the shootings at Virginia Tech in 2007 had been briefly hospitalized on an involuntary commitment and had been released with a community treatment order requiring that he go to outpatient care. He never went.

Marsha confirmed that Delaware patients often don't follow up with treatment, even with the threat of arrest. She added, "We had people disappear all the time. Sometimes we never saw them again. A court order for outpatient commitment is not a guarantee that someone will get treatment at all."

She also noted that outpatient commitment gave family members influence over a patient's care that was not necessarily about the best interest of the patient.

"I would see parents insist a patient need[ed] to be on a commitment order. They'd tell the doctor, 'If you don't put him on an order, I'll sue you,' and they'd get very insistent. So the doctors felt compelled to use orders even if they didn't agree it was necessary. The doctor would say, 'What if the patient does something bad, and I get sued for it?' They were afraid of risking this."

In Texas, the implementation of outpatient commitment is fairly new. One psychiatrist who asked not to be identified mentioned some difficulties with the program. It is being overseen by a group of judges who are invested in making it work. The psychiatrist found that this investment had led to some intrusion in the process: the judges culled through the lists of involuntary patients and handpicked those they felt were likely to succeed with outpatient commitment. They didn't always approve its use with the patients the doctors wanted to see mandated to care. In addition, the judges sometimes requested a level of care that the psychiatrists did not feel was appropriate, including daily visits.

"If the patient says they missed a single medication dose, the judge might say, 'This is why they need to be seen every day.' It puts the doctor in the role of a probation officer!"

It's unusual to have the judiciary steering the medical treatment for patients, and in this case, there have been tensions.

In Washington, DC, a mental health commission convenes twice a week, and every candidate for commitment is seen by the commission, which consists of a judge, a psychiatrist, and a psychologist. The commission can recommend inpatient commitment, outpatient commitment, or release. The patient may challenge a decision and request a jury trial.

Dr. Glenn Miller is a psychiatrist in private practice who sits on the commission, and he said that it is more common to mandate people to outpatient care than to the hospital. Nevertheless, he couldn't offer an opinion about the efficacy of the process. "There is no regular follow-up. We see them at the commission, and we don't see them after. My impression is that they get more intensive services and that they do better."

Dr. E. Fuller Torrey discussed his own experiences with outpatient commitment in the District of Columbia. He found it to be helpful in preventing readmission and allowing patients to live in the community.

I had a patient who had been hospitalized 21 times, and I went to court and told the judge, "Your Honor, I want to release this guy on Friday on the condition that he has to come back every two weeks and get his Haldol shot." The guy would come and say he was only coming because I was making him, and I'd say, "Absolutely!" But it really worked. Even though the patients didn't know they were sick, somehow what I was doing conveyed that I was trying to protect them or trying to help them. But I was surprised that nobody slugged me.

Torrey's Treatment Advocacy Center has been instrumental in getting states to pass outpatient commitment legislation. "One percent of people with severe mental illness should be on involuntary ongoing treatment because they are dangerous," Torrey asserted. "It's a small, but important, number."

In California, outpatient commitment was passed by the state in 2002 as Laura's Law, named for a 19-year-old woman who was killed by a mentally ill man at a mental health center in Nevada County. While the law has been implemented in that county, the area is rural and the number of patients is low; in 2012, California reported that 15 people were on outpatient commitment orders. In May 2014, Orange County also adopted outpatient commitment, but as of this writing, implementation is in the early stages.

Dr. Adam Nelson is a psychiatrist in Mill Valley, California, not far from San Francisco. He's a member of the California Mental Health Planning Council and noted that most mental health services are administered at the county level.

"The medical directors in the state are not in favor of this," Nelson said. "It costs a fortune, and everyone agrees that the counties then have to really beef up the infrastructure for case management and social services. And there's no way to enforce it."

Proponents of the law argue that in Nevada County, outpatient commitment has saved money and that there are provisions for funding through Proposition 63, a millionaire's tax that specifically funds mental health treatment. Nelson said that psychiatrists in California remain skeptical, and there is concern about taking Proposition 63 money from existing programs.

Nelson's thoughts on forced care echoed those of many people I spoke with. "You're not going to get patients to take medications unless they trust you. Everyone may have the best of intentions, but if you drag someone to a place, then hand them a bunch of pills, they may get agitated and combative and end up being injected. And then the damage is done." He also noted that it's essential to provide housing to those with severe mental illnesses. "If people could get supportive housing, they'd be more likely to manage their medications."

While Nelson sees the problems with involuntary care, he personally is in favor of outpatient commitment in California; he sees it as a way to get care for very sick people who can't access it otherwise.

Eleanor lived in California, but her single episode of mania would not have made her eligible for outpatient commitment, even if Laura's Law were implemented in her county. During her hospitalization, however, Dr. Green applied for temporary conservatorship, which would have allowed for another 30 days of hospitalization. The public defender's office appointed an attorney for Eleanor, and a hearing date was set. As it turned out, she was discharged on that date, and the hearing never happened. Nelson noted that conservatorship in California can potentially be extended for two years; although it's about inpatient commitment, it had been standard procedure to drop the conservatorship status when a patient was released from the hospital, but now that is not necessarily happening.

"Suddenly," Nelson said, "people are becoming 'conserved' for longer. Our debate over Laura's Law has caused a consciousness raising. People on conservatorship really struggle because of their illnesses, and a public guardian can help them get services."

As these interviews illustrate, psychiatrists' opinions about the utility of outpatient commitment cover the entire spectrum. In the early days of outpatient commitment, people were more optimistic, due to a limited number of retrospective studies that showed reduced hospitalization rates, shorter lengths of stay, and better compliance with treatment. More recent research has shown less promising results, but the research on outpatient commitment is still limited. Of 7,356 papers written about outpatient commitment, only 2 used the gold-standard methodology of the randomized, controlled trial.

The first was a pilot study done at Bellevue Hospital in New York. Patients were discharged from the hospital and randomly assigned either to court-ordered treatment, which included enhanced services, or to a voluntary program with similar services. There were no significant differences between the two groups on any outcome measure, including rehospitalization, arrests, quality of life, symptomatology, treatment noncompliance, and perceived level of coercion. The dropout rate for the committed patients was high, more than 40 percent, but no noncompliant person was ever taken into custody. The authors concluded that improved outcomes were due to the increase in services, not to the existence of a coercive court order, and that legal coercion might not play a significant role in keeping individuals in treatment.

A similar study done in North Carolina assigned involuntarily hospitalized patients randomly either to outpatient commitment or to the usual voluntary outpatient services upon discharge. They were initially committed for 90 days with an option for a 180-day renewal. For patients whose commitments were extended beyond 90 days, there were fewer hospitalizations and more outpatient contacts per month. They were also less likely to become the victims of crime. The dropout rate for the committed patients was not reported but, as in New York, no noncompliant patient was picked up by police.

Both studies have been criticized for not being truly blind. The North Carolina patients whose commitments were extended were chosen by clinicians who obviously knew the patients' legal status. In New York, both patients and clinicians were confused about AOT status. Some members of the control patient group, and their caseworkers, believed that the patients were court-ordered to treatment.

Another criticism of the two studies was that both specifically excluded patients with a history of serious violence. This is important because outpatient commitment has been justified as a means of reducing violence by people with mental illness. There is nothing in either study to suggest that outpatient commitment had an effect on the overall crime rate in each state.

In terms of the cost savings that were attributed to outpatient commitment, the New York study looked at the cost of services used in the years before and after the implementation of the court order, and the costs clearly went down, on average, for patients who were court-ordered to treatment. The cost savings in New York, however, did not take into account the $125 million that the state pumped into its mental health infrastructure in creating the services these patients used. In a 2009 paper by Swartz, Swanson, Steadman, and Monahan, the researchers were careful to say that the findings might not generalize to other states. Their study also noted that while patients benefited on many measures, only 27 percent of the patients endorsed outpatient commitment after one year.

In another study, Swartz and Swanson looked at the effect of outpatient commitment on cost savings in a group of patients in North Carolina, where no extra funding was provided by the state. For those placed on outpatient commitment for six months or less, the cost for the study group was several thousand dollars higher; it was not until patients were treated on outpatient civil commitment for more than six months that costs began to drop. One might wonder how much the cost savings for 47 patients in rural North Carolina generalize to the rest of the country, but this small study is used to support the idea that involuntary outpatient treatment is cost-effective; furthermore, the data published in 2013 were based on a trial conducted in the 1990s.

Cost savings will be hard to realize because states also have to defend the legality of each provision of outpatient commitment laws, including the requirement to provide community services. In Delaware, where Marsha was committed, the US Department of Justice appointed psychologist Robert Bernstein as the court monitor of a consent decree after an investigation of the Delaware Psychiatric Center, where Marsha was held. The state was accused of violating the Americans with Disabilities Act for failing to provide enough outpatient housing to people with mental illness at risk of hospitalization.

The state of Delaware could be sued for a lack of outpatient services because of a 1999 US Supreme Court case, *Olmstead v. L.C.* This case involved two voluntarily admitted psychiatric patients who sued the state of Georgia for failing to provide the community services that would have allowed them to be released from the hospital. Their doctors agreed that they no longer needed hospitalization, but there weren't sufficient community resources, such as housing and outpatient clinics, to support them if discharged. They filed suit under Title II of the Americans with Disabilities Act, which prohibits states from discriminating against people with disabilities by excluding them from state programs, services, and activities. The patients prevailed, and the Supreme Court held that a lack of funding was not a valid reason to keep disabled people institutionalized when they could otherwise live in the community.

Bernstein described additional problems with outpatient commitment. "Delaware is interesting in that most states have outpatient commitment on the books, and they don't use it. In Delaware, it's a matter of convenience. Physicians see it as a painless way of shielding themselves from liability. And the orders are vague. They simply order someone to go to an outpatient center. It was a total train wreck."

It was quite difficult to figure out how many people were on outpatient commitment in Delaware. NRI Analytics reported that the state had 4,510 patients on orders in 2012, more than any other state and a shockingly high number for a state with a total population of under a million. Bernstein said that this figure just couldn't be right; in September 2011, around the time of the settlement with the Department of Justice, the maximum number of patients was recorded at just under 400, and by June 2014 that number was down to 121. Others told me that no accurate records had been kept. Bernstein observed that since the consent decree, there had been more supported housing in the state, and the outpatient commitment rates had dropped by 55 percent. Inpatient commitment rates had dropped as well.

In spite of the fact that Marsha did well on outpatient commitment and benefited from the treatment she received over time, she joined a group that tried to eliminate its use in Delaware. Outpatient commitment is unlikely to disappear entirely, however.

In 2013 and again in 2015, Congressman Tim Murphy (R-Pa.) proposed federal legislation to fix a broken mental health system, the Helping Families in Mental Health Crisis Act. The first version of the bill required all states to adopt legislation to allow outpatient commitment, or face financial sanctions. When this bill failed, a later version did not include the same mandate for assisted outpatient treatment, but instead provided for financial incentives to states that adopted it. The 2015 version also created a federal database program, called the National Mental Health Policy Laboratory, which must collect state outcome data on individuals with serious mental illness who participate in assisted outpatient treatment. As of this writing, the bill is still awaiting congressional action.

We think it's important to note that while some individuals have benefited from outpatient commitment, it has not been a panacea for society's woes and is not the answer to violent crime. Services—including costly, intensive treatments and housing, case management, and outreach programs—need to be available to the sickest members of society without a court order. For patients who aren't sure if they want care, a treatment team may well need to work to engage them and gain their trust, just as in any field of medicine. Yes, it's easier to mandate care, and perhaps there are times when that's the only way. But if we are going to condone outpatient civil commitment, it needs to be restricted to those patients who have been repeatedly offered comprehensive, kind treatment, without which they repeatedly decompensate only to end up in hospitals and jails. It needs to be limited to patients for whom treatment has been proven to be both effective and tolerable, and it must come with the services that obligate society to the best interests of the individual patient. Forced care in psychiatry has no role as an automatic substitute for the thoughtful engagement of patients in their own treatment.

In a lecture at Sheppard Pratt in February 2014, researcher Jeffrey Swanson concluded:

> Outpatient commitment is neither a cure-all nor a catastrophe. It brings neither an end to violence nor an end to civil rights. It does not affect the majority of people with some form of psychiatric illness. It cannot fix a fiscal crisis of the state in which resources for mental health services continue to shrink. But it may be a reasonable and measured policy that can make effective treatment much more consistently available to those few among us who are most in need of treatment in the community, who at times may actually want it, but in the real world may not get it any other way.

17   Jack Lesser and Mental Health Courts

Jan (not her real name) had been in jail for a number of weeks for missing a half dozen mental health appointments. She was acting strangely prior to being sent to jail and was doing better now. The mental health court's multidisciplinary team, headed by Judge Jack Lesser, noted that her antipsychotic medication had been changed in jail.

"Maybe this medicine is working better. Or maybe she wasn't taking her medication in the community," one of the team members speculated.

"Could she be on a long-acting injection?" a social worker asked.

Another team member pointed out, "She'd have to agree to it; otherwise, the psychiatrist won't give it." To which someone else noted that Jan had once had a bad reaction to a long-acting injectable antipsychotic medication, but that was a different medication than what she was currently taking.

Mental health court (MHC) is a unique setting. Acting as a medical team isn't a traditional role of courts, nor are care coordination and decisions regarding treatment options. In mental health courts, it's the judge, and not a treating physician, who orders defendants to different treatment programs based on the recommendations of the team.

People come to MHCs after they have been arrested. These courts are voluntary; arrestees are offered the option of going to an MHC as an alternative to incarceration. If they don't want treatment, they can simply refuse participation and elect to go through the court system to be tried for the crime for which they are charged.

This book focuses on civil commitment, a process used for people who have not been legally charged with committing crimes. The issue of coerced care for criminal defendants evokes a bit less angst among many members of US society. Although MHCs are voluntary, this chapter is included because, in our view, they may be part of the solution to many of the issues that advocates hope to fix by forcing treatment.

Those in favor of involuntary care, and particularly those in favor of outpatient civil commitment, believe that wider use of involuntary treatment might prevent people from committing crimes in the first place, but they also acknowledge that mental health courts might keep people out of jails and prisons. MHCs are a way to funnel people out of bad places—jails, shelters, sleeping on the streets—and into appropriate services, and so they deserve a place in this book.

I visited a mental health court on a Monday in January 2015. The presiding judge was Jack Lesser, a slim, soft-spoken gentleman who is not at all intimidating, but rumor has it that he will sentence you to 10 years with a smile on his face; he has a reputation for being tough on criminals. The Baltimore City Mental Health Court is based in the John R. Hargrove Sr. Building. The Hargrove courthouse is a modern, two-story structure made of cement and green glass; it sticks out on East Patapsco Avenue because of its newness in a section of Baltimore that can be described only as weary and dilapidated.

"I look at mental health court defendants differently than I do a regular criminal case," Lesser said. "While I don't make up my mind until I hear the specifics in any case, and I always keep an open mind, if you're on regular probation with me and you violate, there's a good possibility that you're going to end up in jail. But not so much in mental health court; it depends on what everyone else on the team has to say about the person. I'm hearing from a lot of different people, a lot of different views, and that all factors into what I'm ultimately going to decide."

Lesser has a soft spot for the underdog. He was quick to note that he was the first in his family to finish high school, much less go to college and law school. His older brother suffered from educational disabilities and felt more like a younger brother to him. As an adult, the judge's brother was diagnosed with bipolar disorder. He was able to work, but he required a good deal of supervision.

"Sitting in mental health court has given me a much better understanding of mental illness. It's made it easier for me to spot a potential issue in court if someone's acting not quite right, whereas before I might wonder: why are they being so rude or using profane language in the courtroom? I guess because of my brother, it's been a good learning experience for me. Do people with mental illnesses get a little more sympathy from me? Absolutely."

In his book, *Crazy: A Father's Search through America's Mental Health Madness*, Pete Earley described the chaos of the Florida judicial system. There, a mentally ill defendant charged with a minor offense, such as trespassing, could be sent to a forensic hospital to be made competent to stand trial. After months of hospitalization, the defendant would be returned to jail for a hearing, but while awaiting that hearing he or she would not be given medications and might become incompetent again. The person would then be returned to the hospital for treatment. This resulted in a cycle of incarceration in a variety of facilities.

In Baltimore, the situation was fortunately not as bad as the system Earley described. Newly arrested prisoners were screened for medical and mental health disorders when they arrived at the booking facility, and those charged with misdemeanor offenses who also had psychiatric disorders were often referred to the city's long-standing pretrial diversion program, the Forensic Alternative Services Team (FAST). The term "pretrial diversion" means that the defendant is contacted and interviewed before any hearing that might determine guilt or innocence.

FAST reviews the defendant's legal and psychiatric history, then sets up a community treatment plan. If the person agrees to the treatment plan, the FAST social worker appears in court with the defendant and presents the plan. If the judge agrees with the proposed treatment, the defendant can be released on probation, provided either he pleads guilty or is convicted of the crime.

Depending on the charge, the person may be eligible for deferred adjudication, also called "probation before judgment." When this happens, the defendant is placed directly on probation, and no verdict is entered on the record. If people with mental illness successfully complete probation, they are legally able to say that they have never been convicted of a crime. Finally, the third possible outcome is that the charge is dropped completely (*nolle prossed*, a Latin term meaning "not prosecuted").

Unlike most court hearings, where one side is pitted against the other, a mental health court is nonadversarial. It's a type of specialty court known as a "problem-solving court." In other words, there is a hearing where both sides come together as a team to fix a problem, usually a social problem involving a particular issue, and the goal is treatment rather than punishment. Drug courts are one example of a problem-solving court. For mental health courts, the goal is to solve the problem of people with serious mental illnesses who are caught up in the criminal justice system. The docket for mental health courts is much smaller than the docket for other courts and typically includes 15 cases in an afternoon. In contrast, other courts, like those for serious traffic or domestic violence incidents, may hear 30–50 cases, or more, in the same few hours.

On the morning of my visit, before court began, the full team met in the judge's library on the second floor, and Lesser was briefed on the status of all the cases he would hear that day. All sides were present in the room: the state's attorney (the prosecution), the public defender, social workers with the FAST program, and the defendant's probation officer. The morning meeting—which is held for no other court—felt more like a psychiatric team meeting than a legal proceeding. People went around the table and gave input about how defendants were doing, including what the counselors at their residential facilities and day programs said about their behavior and progress, whether they were making it to their appointments and taking their medications, what their psychiatrists and therapists said about their participation in treatment, and, perhaps most important, what their mothers had to say.

There was a level of investment by court personnel that is not seen with other defendants, and care was coordinated with an effort that is usually seen in medical, but not legal, settings. It reminded me of Dr. DePaulo conducting morning rounds in the hospital.

Lesser started sitting in mental health court nearly a decade ago at the request of Judge Charlotte Cooksey. The Baltimore City Mental Health Court was started by Cooksey in 2002, and she presided until her retirement in 2008. Cooksey came to her position with an interest in mental health; she had worked as a counselor in a mental health facility during college and law school, and like Lesser, she had a sibling with a psychiatric disorder—a brother with schizophrenia. She told me:

I began noticing what was apparent nationwide. Psychiatrically ill people were coming into the criminal justice system in large numbers. We saw people who were not competent to stand trial and had to manage the procedure piecemeal, and there was no one whose responsibility it was to follow that case. Some people came to the courts over and over again; the typical way of handling a criminal case was just not adequate for this type of defendant. Back then, problem-solving courts were just getting started in Maryland, and our administrative judge agreed to give it a try.

Cooksey visited mental health courts in other states, including New York, Washington, and Florida. "We took back the best of what we saw in these programs."

One of the sites that Cooksey visited was the first mental health court, which opened in June 1997 in Broward County, Florida. Three others quickly followed in Washington, California, and Alaska. In 2003 there were 90 programs nationwide, and according to the Council of State Governments, by 2009 there were more than 200 mental health courts. The courts were popular with advocates for the mentally ill, and funding from the federal government provided an additional impetus.

In 2000, Congress had passed the America's Law Enforcement and Mental Health Project act, which provided technical assistance and funding for the creation of mental health courts. The act required the coordinated delivery of services, voluntary participation, training of law enforcement and the judiciary, and the ongoing supervision of offenders. In 2004, the Mentally Ill Offender Treatment and Crime Reduction Act authorized an additional $50 million in initiatives to coordinate care between the criminal justice and public mental health systems.

The Baltimore City Mental Health Court started as a way to consolidate all the cases involving the mentally ill onto a single docket, overseen and tracked by a single judge. The mental health court docket came to include FAST program defendants, defendants referred for competency assessments, and mental health court defendants.

"Everyone who comes into the jail system is screened for mental health issues," Lesser explained. "So if they see someone with a mental health issue, they might call the FAST representative to come see them. Also during bail reviews, if someone's acting inappropriately, I might say I want FAST to interview this person to see if there are any mental health issues.

Another way is from a regular criminal docket, and I've done that myself many times if they are exhibiting behavior that's not appropriate in the courtroom and I think there's something wrong."

Compared to other states, where the wait to transfer to a hospital can be several months long, in Maryland defendants may be transferred to a state hospital within days. When the patient returns from the hospital, treatment information is sent to the jail so care can be continued.

In fiscal year 2011, the mental health court in Baltimore heard approximately 340 cases. Competency evaluations were ordered in 128 cases, and 11 cases involved pleas of not criminally responsible, in other words, an insanity defense. In addition, 102 voluntary defendants entered the program. This is a tiny fraction of all criminal cases heard in the city of Baltimore; on any given day as many as 350 people may be arrested. It's hard to imagine there aren't people who would benefit from MHC but who never get offered the option of participating.

Even with an active mental health court and several points for screening and entry, the Baltimore correctional system still has many inmates with serious psychiatric disorders who are receiving treatment from the jails' mental health services. Some people never get offered mental health court and stay in jail because the charge is too serious. No one would want a person back on the streets—even a very ill person—who had been arrested for murder, rape, or kidnapping. Another reason some people do not go to the MHC is because those who are innocent would never have a chance to challenge the charge or dispute the evidence against them, since there is no actual trial. For an innocent person, an acquittal may be more important than an offer of treatment.

Cooksey noted that the most common charge for a mental health court defendant was assault. She added that there were several crimes that disqualify a defendant from being diverted to MHC, including domestic violence crimes or a past conviction for murder, rape, abduction, armed robbery, carjacking, or a sexual offense. Participation comes at a cost: the defendant pleads guilty and agrees to comply with the recommendations of the court, which may include requirements for mental health treatment (therapy and medications), participation in psychosocial or vocational rehabilitative programs, substance abuse treatment and testing, and living in supervised housing. Any failure to meet these obligations is addressed in the courtroom and may include increased supervision or a jail sentence.

While the purpose of MHC is to keep people out of jail and get them into treatment, it doesn't always succeed.

"You don't want very ill people in jail," Cooksey said. "They don't follow rules well, and they end up serving their whole sentences because they can't get reduced time for credit for participating in some of the rehabilitative programs, which often won't take people on medications, much less psychiatric medications."

Every case may not be a success, but what about mental health courts in general? Are these programs effective? Do they keep mentally ill people out of jail?

The theory of "transinstitutionalization," also known as the Penrose hypothesis, has not yet been proven and remains controversial. The relationship among the number of available hospital beds, the size of correctional systems, and the number of mentally ill people within them is a complex dynamic between economic and legal forces, as our exploration of the mental health court process revealed.

Outcome studies of MHCs are difficult to do well since the participants aren't randomly chosen and violent offenders are often excluded. Nevertheless, some studies suggest that mental health court participants tend to re-offend less frequently, are charged with less severe crimes at re-arrest, and take longer to re-offend.

Participation in a mental health court may also reduce the risk of violence. In one prospective study, 88 jail detainees enrolled in MHC were compared to 81 detainees who were managed through the usual court procedures. They were all followed for one year, and their arrest records were reviewed. MHC participants were significantly less likely to commit a violent act than those not involved in the program. Even though most were originally charged with felonies, only 25 percent of the MHC participants perpetrated a violent crime within the year, compared to 42 percent of those who did not go through mental health court. Furthermore, a four-site study funded by the MacArthur Foundation found preliminary evidence that mental health court supervision was associated with positive outcomes in several categories, including lower criminal recidivism rates and increased treatment engagement.

Exactly how MHC benefits an offender isn't clear. We would like to think that mental health intervention and treatment are the key to rehabilitation, but other factors associated with court supervision may also play a role. Frequent status hearings, close communication between the court and treatment providers, immediate consequences for noncompliance, and even the nature of the judge-patient relationship may help make the programs work.

You would think that with results like this, there would be even more mental health court programs popping up around the United States. And while it's true that more are being funded, the cost savings have not yet been realized. While the costs of incarceration are significant, MHC diversion shifts the expense to the community. The price for the average MHC participant is about $4,000 more per person in government funding, compared to those who remain in the criminal justice system, due to the need for additional community services. Even considering the reduced length of time in jail and fewer criminal prosecutions, MHCs are a zero-sum game economically, at least in the first year. It is possible that the economic benefits of mental health courts show up later, since recovery is a long-term process. But maybe the main value of MHC is not found in its economics. Recovery, rehabilitation, and success at keeping people from re-offending cannot be measured in dollars.

"So why does a judge come into mental health court? Because you want to help someone turn their life around," Lesser explained.

Maybe they've been coming through the system for years, maybe because they've been using drugs, or because they have an underlying mental illness and no one's ever treated it, so they continue to come through the system without treatment. They go in the door, out the door, and go back to their same lifestyle without anything ever changing, while the taxpayers are paying more and more money. Instead, you have them come into mental health court and get the treatment they've needed for all these years, perhaps getting them to stop using drugs for the rest of their lives, perhaps get[ting] them to find a job and a stable living. Everybody feels good about it when someone is successful.

When a defendant is doing well, the feeling in the court is celebratory, unlike a typical judicial setting.

"Congratulations to you," Lesser told one defendant. "That's a wonderful report." There are kudos all around, and periodically there are certificates of acknowledgment that he reads aloud. "This is in recognition of your continued efforts and compliance. Keep up the good work."

Every few months, the court holds a graduation ceremony for people who have completed their time with the MHC successfully. Food is served, and the defendants bring their families. It's a creative twist on a criminal arrest: the sentence gets framed as a personal accomplishment rather than as a reason for shame and disgrace.

Cooksey said, "You get to see people get better, and you relate to people in an entirely different way. I loved getting to see the cases from beginning to end, and I liked getting to know the families. It seemed to have made a difference and to improve the quality of their lives."

Hidaya Hamilton is a parole and probation officer for the Baltimore court, and she explained how her work differs from that of a typical probation officer. "I meet with our probationers either weekly or biweekly, depending on the amount of time they have been on probation. We are constantly in communication with their treatment providers. We are often involved in the enhancement of treatment plans, if necessary and if it's determined to be clinically appropriate in order to keep the probationer in compliance." Her caseload consists of 30–35 active cases, in contrast to the caseload of 200 or more for a probation officer who is not in a specialty court.

Hamilton's supervisor, Evelyn Young, told me:

> We go in the homes, assisted living, group homes, hospitals, and psych wards, and we ask family members and providers questions. We scope out the living quarters for client safety and compliance. We visit the treatment programs, day programs, or other facilities, and we have face-to-face team meetings with them. We are the eyes and ears for the court. We are the ones on the mental health court team that get out there in the communities, and they are tough communities. On top of that, we still have to provide written reports to the court one to two times per week and to perform other office duties on demand.

When it was Jan's turn before Judge Lesser in mental health court on the afternoon of my observation, she appeared in a pink jumpsuit and handcuffs.

"Had enough of jail?" Lesser asked her. She'd been in for three weeks for violating the terms of her probation repeatedly.

"Yes, Your Honor."

"You understand that you have to keep your appointments?"

"I do. And they talked to me about taking an injection, and I'm fine with that," she volunteered.

Ultimately, her psychiatrist would need to agree that this was medically appropriate. At times, court-ordered treatments can be problematic if the needed resources don't exist or if the treating physician believes that what the judge has ordered is not what is medically indicated. Jan's release from jail was arranged for the next day.

Todd (not his real name) had a more complicated story. He was ready to graduate from MHC after several years of monitored treatment. He'd gone to his appointments and taken the medications, but in recent months there had been a number of positive drug screens. In addition, he'd never paid the restitution for the property he destroyed during his original offense. The restitution, Judge Lesser asserted, was not the issue, but the drug use was. Years into treatment, the prosecution was recommending that Todd serve the full sentence for his crime, months in jail. It was a property crime, Todd's only arrest, and not one that he would have served time for if he'd gone through criminal proceedings. Mental health court had funneled him into treatment, but he needed to abstain from drug use as one of its conditions. The public defender made the case in the morning meeting with Lesser that Todd had gone to every appointment, had taken medications as instructed, and had no arrests in the years he was in mental health court.

Todd insisted that the drug test was wrong. "Your Honor, I don't want to go to jail. I didn't do anything."

He was sentenced to four months—half the time the prosecution had recommended—and escorted out in handcuffs. All cases don't have happy endings, and this was a case no one felt good about. Todd might have come out better—at least in terms of time spent in jail for this particular crime—if he'd refused the offer to move to mental health court, but he may well have continued being quite ill with a psychotic disorder that, before his arrest, had never been diagnosed or treated.

"Being a judge can be a very depressing job on a daily basis," Lesser said. "We see so many people who come through regular criminal courts and they have had all these tragedies that occur during their lives, and as a result it's led them to a life of drugs. And we see mostly drug cases at the district level in Baltimore City; in some fashion, almost all crimes are related to drugs. It could be shoplifting, it could be prostitution, but you don't have the services available to a regular criminal defendant that you have in mental health court."

Mental health court is not the only answer to the problem of involuntary treatment, and it may not even be the best answer for a particular person, but it does address one enormous problem that comes with insisting that patients get involuntary care. In the case of patients who are treated involuntarily on *civil* commitments, people are denied liberty and confined to a hospital because they might be dangerous to themselves or others. Ordering people to treatment because they *might* commit a dangerous act can be problematic; it means that people lose their freedom based on a prediction that could very well be wrong. Although used in the name of protecting innocent people from the dangers of the mentally ill, it casts a wide net, denying civil rights to many people who will never harm anyone. At the same time, if someone is clearly suffering from a psychotic illness and their disorganization has already resulted in criminal behavior, at least the playing field has better definition.

Mental health courts limit their authority to people who already have been charged with a crime, and participation is voluntary. MHCs are not without controversy, however; some people believe that this intervention comes too late, after a crime has already been committed. Others believe that mental health courts don't extend far enough and that participation should be mandatory even for those charged with minor, nonviolent offenses. Still others believe that MHCs are being misused to manage nuisance behavior by mentally ill people who normally would not be arrested.

As with most of the interventions we've discussed, mental health courts require community services, and community services come with a price tag.

So, is mental health court worth it?

"I'm going to say yes," Judge Lesser said, "because if you're able to help even one person, there's one less defendant in the system. If you spend the money now to treat someone, and they become a productive member of society, then it's a good thing."

Sociologist Henry Steadman, who heads a New York–based policy research group, noted that it is important to view the numbers in context.

"We have taken a hard-core, challenging population that has failed repeatedly in all three systems: criminal justice, substance abuse and mental health," Steadman said on MPR News, "and has cycled and is a particularly challenging group, and we have come up with an intervention that is a 20 to 25 percent improvement on almost all the measures. My evaluation is that's pretty damn good in today's world."

Six

A DANGER TO SELF OR OTHERS

People with mental health problems are almost never dangerous. In fact, they are more likely to be the victims than the perpetrators. At the same time, mental illness has been the common denominator in one act of mass violence after another.

—Senator Roy Blunt (R-Mo.)

Tiburon, California, in Marin County, is a half-hour drive from the Golden Gate Bridge. Tiburon is a stunning and peaceful town with houses etched into the mountains overlooking the San Francisco Bay. Tiburon is a high-rent district with no shortage of shops or restaurants. It is a safe place to live, and Dan (not his real name) would likely have remained safe even if he hadn't owned a gun, but still, it is a US citizen's right to possess one.

As sensitive as it was to recruit people to talk about involuntary psychiatric treatment, it proved even harder to find anyone who would talk about guns and mental illness. I contacted a representative of the Associated Gun Clubs of Baltimore. He had fired one of his own physicians for lecturing him about gun safety, and he didn't think any of the club's members would be willing to talk. Doctors, he noted, are seen by gun owners as an extension of the government. Internet message boards also proved to be unhelpful when it came to looking for a story about guns and mental illness. People were happy to engage in casual conversation, but before they would speak in depth, they wanted reassurance that we were not in favor of gun control, regardless of whether that was relevant to the topic of this book.

Eventually, our police contacts provided us with a story. The report is in the public domain but, as psychiatrists, we wanted to protect the patient's privacy, so we changed the demographic details. As beautiful as Tiburon is, Dan doesn't actually live there.

Dan had been hospitalized for a psychiatric problem years before, when he was in the military. At that time, he was acting strangely and was committed to the hospital involuntarily. Following his release, he was honorably discharged from the military. Anyone who has been involuntarily admitted in California is ineligible to legally purchase a gun there, but Dan's hospitalization was in another state, and it was decades before these records were computerized.

After his discharge, Dan sought help and continued to see a therapist for years. For the most part, things went well until early in 2012, when something changed. Dan started to accuse people of unusual and violent acts that could not be substantiated. He abruptly stopped seeing his therapist because he was convinced that the therapist was part of a group conspiring against him. Dan had medication to treat delusions, but no one knew if he was taking it, not even his wife. He became angry, erratic, and disorganized in his thoughts. Soon, his job was in danger.

Dan's behavior became even stranger in the spring of 2012. He went into a gun store to purchase a handgun. In spite of his military background, he asked the clerk if the gun he wanted could kill someone. The clerk assured him that it could, then sold him the firearm. Dan returned to the store a few days later. He wanted to return the revolver and get his money back, but the best the clerk could offer was store credit, and that was not good enough.

Dan left with his gun and went to a local police station with the intent of donating the firearm to charity. While the police don't serve as a station for charitable gun contributions, they did agree to take the revolver and melt it down. Dan left the gun with the police, but he still wasn't satisfied and called the precinct often—sometimes, several times a day—to ask if the revolver had been destroyed yet. He was told that there was a process to do this, and the process was moving along. Dan accused the police of having lost his gun, and he submitted the necessary paperwork to have the firearm returned to him. This triggered an investigation by the firearms unit.

An agent at the unit contacted Dan's employer and learned that Dan would go for long periods without communicating with his co-workers. At times, he'd lock himself in his office and not answer the door or the phone, or he would repeatedly slam the door. Interviews with his family and therapist confirmed the suspicion that he had lapsed into a state of psychosis, and a decision was made to bring Dan in for a psychiatric evaluation.

On the morning of August 6, weeks after Dan had asked the gun store clerk if the revolver he bought could kill a person, police officers waited for Dan outside his home. They had been instructed to bring in a "mentally deranged suspect" on a 5150, California's term for an involuntary psychiatric admission.

Dan would have none of it, and he wasn't going peacefully. He managed to break free of the officers' attempts to restrain him, and, when things got hectic, a police officer attempted to stun Dan with a Taser. This proved to be ineffective: one of the electrodes went into Dan's tie, while others missed him or just didn't work. While everyone struggled, Dan yelled religious chants and struck the two police officers. He was eventually restrained and brought in, but both officers required treatment for lacerations and contusions.

While it may seem obvious that people with mental illnesses should not own firearms, it's not as though the presence or absence of a psychiatric illness is a constant thing—symptoms can come and go. People can have chronic illnesses, they can have intermittent illnesses, or a psychiatric episode can be a one-time event, as it was for Eleanor. In fact, community surveys show that nearly half of Americans will suffer from at least one episode of mental illness at some point during their lives.

Most psychiatric symptoms don't cause people to be dangerous or unsafe with firearms, and people with psychiatric disorders don't wear signs indicating that they suffer from these problems. Some illnesses are well controlled with medications, others remit spontaneously, and some people have constant symptoms, either because they won't take medications or because the medications don't work well for them. The medical profession's ability to come up with an accurate prognosis is far from perfect, and many variables affect the likelihood of a good outcome, including how people functioned before they became ill, their access to treatment, their social circumstances, and whether they also have problems with drugs and alcohol. The diagnosis, which we don't always get right and which may change over time, is only one clue as to how a patient will do.

So while we might all agree that mentally unstable people should not have easy access to firearms, we don't have a way of defining who exactly those mentally unstable people are.

On July 24, 2012, days after the fatal theater shooting in Aurora, Colorado, President Barack Obama made the following statement, "I believe the majority of gun owners would agree that we should do everything possible to prevent criminals and fugitives from purchasing weapons; that we should check someone's criminal record before they can check out a gun seller; that a mentally unbalanced individual should not be able to get his hands on a gun so easily. These steps shouldn't be controversial. They should be common sense."

At that point, no information had been released that indicated that the shooter had a history of a significant mental disorder. He was a graduate student who had sought treatment at his university mental health center; he had never been hospitalized or charged with a violent crime. While he was struggling with a mental illness, there was nothing about his history that would have prevented him from legally purchasing guns. Surely, no one is suggesting that all college students who go to a mental health clinic should then be banned from owning a gun. It's much easier to determine that someone is dangerous after they've killed a group of strangers.

We later learned that the Aurora shooter had talked of wanting to kill people. It may well be that a desire to murder is a much better predictor than a blanket diagnosis of "mental illness" that someone would be unsafe with a gun. Or perhaps, unusual patterns of purchasing firearms or ammunition could alert authorities: from May 10 to July 14, 2012, the shooter purchased tear gas grenades online and legally bought nearly 6,300 rounds of ammunition, two .40-caliber Glock pistols, a .223-caliber semiautomatic rifle, a 12-gauge shotgun, protective clothing, laser lights, bomb-making materials, and handcuffs.

When it comes to the topic of firearms and mental illness, the foremost expert is Jeffrey Swanson, a professor in the Department of Psychiatry and Behavioral Sciences at the Duke University School of Medicine. He is quick to point out that he's neither a psychiatrist—which everyone assumes he is—nor a conventional college professor who lectures to undergraduates from a podium. He's a medical sociologist who studies the epidemiology of violence and serious mental illness and the effects of community-based interventions. In his tweed jacket and jeans, he projects a rather debonair persona, and it's not until he really gets started talking about his work that his passion and unsurpassed knowledge overpower his studied calmness.

Swanson discussed how mental illness increases the chance that someone will die by suicide, and firearms are often involved. When it comes to homicide, however, the link with mental illness is both small and far from predictive.

"If we were to look at all firearms deaths from 2001 to 2010, that would be about 306,000 deaths by firearms, and 57 percent of those are suicides," Swanson said.

If we could take out the deaths from mental illness, very little of it would be homicide. If we were to factor out the contribution of serious mental illness to gun deaths, that number would go down by about 100,000. But 95 percent of the reduction would come from reducing suicide. Very little of it would come from reducing homicide, because homicide is a problem that doesn't have a whole lot to do with mental illness. Most people with mental illness aren't violent, and there aren't that many people in the general population who are seriously mentally ill.

Because guns are such lethal implements for suicide, Swanson does believe that firearms should be taken from people who are in the midst of a mental health crisis.

In Florida, we're doing this study where we're looking at cases where people have already committed suicide. So we've found 50 people who were receiving services under the public behavioral health care system; they had serious mental illnesses, and 80 percent of them were able to go buy a gun legally; they weren't disqualified. Think about the circumstances and the loss of hope and the people left behind. Some of these were probably impulsive acts of intoxicated young people who, if they had tried some other means, they might have survived, but you're not going to survive a gunshot to the brain.

Legislators, he believes, should be focusing on aspects other than mental health when it comes to preventing homicides.

"Past violence remains the single biggest predictor of future violence.

Any history of violent behavior is a much stronger predictor of future violence than a mental health diagnosis."

He talked about a study he did with Ron Kessler at Harvard. They used national survey data to estimate the number of people with impulsive angry behavior who also have access to firearms. "These are people who get explosively angry. They smash and break things and get into physical fights. And they have guns. We're just going to figure that that's a bad combination."

Swanson noted that angry people with guns do have a fair amount of psychopathology—not major mental illnesses like schizophrenia, but personality disorders, intermittent explosive disorder, posttraumatic stress disorder, alcoholism, or some component of anxiety.

> So you can say that many of them have mental health problems, but they are not the kinds of disorders that are common in people who get involuntarily committed and lose their gun rights. Less than 10 percent of them will ever have been hospitalized for a mental health problem. What this means is that the vast majority of this ostensibly scary group of people are never going to be exposed to a disqualifying mental health adjudication. If we want to think about modifying [the] risk of gun violence, we need to do it in a very different way.

Swanson suggested using behavioral indicators, rather than mental health diagnoses, to disqualify people for gun ownership. Misdemeanor assaults, drug and alcohol problems, driving under the influence—these are things he believes should disqualify people from owning guns.

It's not that there is no connection at all between psychiatric symptoms and the risk of violence. Swanson has also done studies showing that psychotic symptoms, such as delusions that involve a perceived threat, can increase the risk of interpersonal violence in people with schizophrenia. But even there, other factors often intervene and interact with the psychosis. He discussed a study done in the United Kingdom that looked at the connection between persecutory delusions and violence.

"So if I have a delusional belief that you just poisoned my espresso," Swanson said while we were talking in a coffee shop (where I had certainly not poisoned his espresso), "I am going to be upset at you for doing that, and I may be afraid as well. But if I'm not angry, I'm a lot less likely to do anything about it. It's anger that mediates the relationship between psychosis and violence."

Swanson said that antipsychotic medications decrease violence in people with schizophrenia, but not in the group of people with schizophrenia who were antisocial before they developed schizophrenia.

"You've got these people, all of whom have schizophrenia, and you can split them into two groups with different pathways to violence. One group is violent because of acute psychosis, and they can be treated, and the other group may be violent because they are angry, antisocial people who will still be violent. It's the same thing with crime and mental illness in general. You have to separate out what the primary motivational system is, and this can be very hard."

The possession of guns by psychiatric patients wasn't addressed by law until the federal Gun Control Act of 1968. This law prohibited the ownership of firearms by people who were convicted of certain crimes, addicted to certain drugs, "adjudicated as a mental defective," or committed to a mental institution. This meant that people could not own a gun if they had been legally found to be a danger to themselves or others, or had been found to lack the mental capacity to contract or manage their own affairs. It also banned gun ownership by people who were incompetent to stand trial and by insanity acquittees, even if the crimes they were charged with were minor property offenses rather than crimes of violence. People who were admitted to mental health facilities temporarily for observation or who were voluntarily admitted were excluded from the ban even if the reason for admission was a violent incident. If all this sounds counterintuitive, that's because it is. Gun laws are not written by psychiatrists, and we struggle along with our patients to understand why gun rights remain with some people while they are removed from others.

When the District of Columbia outlawed the possession of handguns in the home, DC police officer Dick Heller sued for the right to keep a weapon for personal protection. He believed that the Second Amendment protected an individual's right to own a gun and that the ban violated that right. Up to this point, the Second Amendment was always interpreted to mean that a state had the right to regulate arms owned by members of a militia—in other words, the right only applied to certain groups of people rather than to any particular individual. In the 2008 landmark case *District of Columbia v. Heller*, the US Supreme Court revisited this principle for the first time since 1939. Justice Antonin Scalia wrote the majority opinion in a way that dramatically broadened access to guns. He held that the Second Amendment applied to each citizen, not to any particular group of people. He was careful to add that certain restrictions on gun ownership were constitutional: the "possession of firearms by felons and the mentally ill."

In 2010, another Supreme Court case, *McDonald v. Chicago*, expanded that opinion to apply to all the states rather than just the District of Columbia. Justice Samuel Alito echoed the opinion of Scalia in the *Heller* case when he wrote, "We made it clear in *Heller* that our holding did not cast doubt on such longstanding regulatory measures as 'prohibitions on the possession of firearms by felons and the mentally ill.' We repeat those assurances here."

Clearly, the justices viewed psychiatric patients as potential threats to public safety. This prohibition isn't permanent, however, and some day the Supreme Court may revisit the issue of gun ownership by people with mental illness.

For example, in December 2014 the Sixth Circuit of the US Court of Appeals, in *Tyler v. Hillsdale County*, found that a history of civil commitment alone was not enough to permanently prohibit someone from buying a gun. Clifford Tyler, 73 years old, had been committed to a psychiatric hospital for less than a month following a devastating divorce in 1986. Tyler's wife had left him for another man and depleted their bank account. His daughters had found him sitting in the middle of the floor at home, pounding his head and crying nonstop. He wasn't sleeping, and he felt suicidal. The daughters called the police, and Tyler was admitted to a psychiatric hospital.

At the commitment hearing, a judge found by clear and convincing evidence that Tyler was mentally ill and that he represented a danger to himself and others. Tyler managed to pass through this crisis, and after his release, he required no treatment for the next 25 years. When he went to buy a firearm in 2011, however, he was told that he couldn't make the purchase because his civil commitment showed up in the FBI's National Instant Criminal Background Check System (NICS). He was unable to challenge the system's data because neither the state nor the federal government provided funding to carry out a gun restoration process that would legally verify that an individual was mentally sound, in other words, no longer a "disqualified person." Tyler sued, and the Sixth Circuit held that without a finding of *present* mental illness and dangerousness, Tyler's Second Amendment right had been violated.

In the year following the Sandy Hook school massacre, nearly every state considered some type of legislation related to gun ownership. New York passed the SAFE Act, a gun control bill that required mental health professionals to report any patient who the clinician felt was "likely to be dangerous." Once reported to NICS, mental health patients could no longer purchase a gun, and if they already owned firearms, they were required to turn them in. States were also pressured to comply with the existing federal requirement to report civilly committed patients. Previously, many states had either failed to do this or had done so inconsistently.

In Maryland, the law before 2013 forbade people from owning a gun if they had been hospitalized on a psychiatric unit for more than 30 consecutive days. The patients' level of dangerousness or their diagnosis was not considered, so psychotic patients who were committed to a hospital for homicidal ideas or violent behavior were not barred from owning a gun if they were released in two weeks. On the other hand, patients who were voluntarily admitted for treatment of an eating disorder and who never presented a danger could not own a firearm if they had remained in a hospital for 31 days.

In 2013, the Maryland law was changed to require the administrative law judge who presided over a civil commitment hearing to order patients to surrender their weapons if they were found to be a danger to others, and also to order patients not to own any weapons in the future until they could prove they were no longer a "disqualified person." Patients also have to be reported to the NICS database. Oddly, the revised law does not require the judge to order the removal of weapons if patients are found to be a danger to themselves.

In California, where both Dan and Eleanor live, the laws regarding gun ownership are more stringent. Anyone held on a 5150—a 72-hour hold for evaluation—for being dangerous loses the right to purchase or possess a gun for five years, even if the patient is released by the judge at the hearing. Eleanor was held on a 5150 for being "gravely disabled," but not for being dangerous. But because she was detained at the hearing, her 5150 was converted to a 5250 for a 14-day detention. After being held on a 5250, Eleanor cannot purchase or own a firearm. She could request a hearing to contest her right to own a gun in California, but it's not clear that this would change her right to own a gun under federal law.

Eleanor has not tried to purchase a firearm.

"As someone who has been hospitalized, I assume I am unable to buy a gun. Even that generalization—that all people who have ever been in a psychiatric hospital should not be able to buy a gun—is flawed, in my opinion. I am quite sane and calm and nonviolent, even though I had a single hospitalization."

In Ohio, where Lily was hospitalized, the probate courts are required to report the names of people who have been committed to psychiatric facilities in order to prevent them from getting conceal-carry permits. In August 2013, a local television station reported that the state's attorney general had said the numbers just weren't adding up and that the probate courts were underreporting. We don't know if Lily could purchase a gun if she tried to do so.

To a certain extent, it makes sense to use civil commitment as a criterion for gun restriction, since there at least is a hearing with a presentation of evidence related to dangerousness, and a requirement to prove danger-ousness by clear and convincing evidence.

Some states, like New York through the SAFE Act, rely on mental health professionals to assess the likelihood of dangerousness using only their clinical judgment. There is no requirement for that opinion to be based on any specific diagnosis, a hospital stay, a violent act, or even known gun ownership. The criterion for reporting is based solely on a mental health professional's best guess, and this creates a few problems.

First, there is the possibility that someone who needs psychiatric care won't seek it for fear of being reported. This phenomenon is known as the "chilling effect." In essence, those who most need help may be afraid to ask for it, and this may create circumstances that make society less safe in the long run. Second, it leaves those with psychiatric disorders as the only group of people who can lose a constitutionally protected civil right based on what is essentially another person's intuition. As of October 2014, under the SAFE Act, 34,500 New Yorkers had been placed in a no-guns database for psychiatric reasons, either because of hospitaliza-tions or because they were assumed to be dangerous. The vast majority of these reports came from hospitals. It's not clear how many, if any, came from therapists notifying the police of patients they believed might be dangerous. And it remains to be seen if any of these reports have had any impact on gun violence in New York.

If no effects are found, this wouldn't be surprising since acts of gun violence are rare among people with mental disorders. As Jeffrey Swanson noted, other factors, such as drug and alcohol use, violent tendencies, early exposure to gun violence, and problems with irritability and anger management, are more predictive of gun violence than is a diagnosis of mental illness. There are many ways in which a person can be destructive, disturbed, and dangerous without being mentally ill.

Dr. Torrey shared his thoughts on guns and mental illness:

> What we're talking about has nothing to do with guns. I understand how the issues get confused. We often end up on gun control because liberals aren't interested in issues of involuntary treatment; they are interested in gun control issues. So the traditional, knee-jerk liberal response to mass shootings is "we need to control guns." I fully agree that we need to control guns; I'm from upstate New York, where people hunt, and you're never going to take all guns away. But [regulating] the kind of clips and number of bullets you can shoot within a given amount of time, it might limit how many people would be killed, but it's not going to stop the shootings. I think it would decrease the kill rate in mass shootings, but I don't think it would have any effect on whether the mass shooting took place or not. In China you have mass knifings, and there are several instances in my book where people drive cars on the sidewalk and kill people. There are lots of ways to kill people. If the voices are telling you to kill people, you'll kill them. I'm a proponent of gun control but for other reasons.

Here is one last aspect of this discussion: there are no laws that forbid household members from owning firearms if they share a residence with very ill or dangerous people. Even if laws could be crafted so that the exact population of people with mental illness who are likely to become violent with a gun could be identified, such legislation would be limited in its efficacy. In the case of the young man who killed 27 people in Newtown, for example, the guns were the legal property of his mother, and neither the shooter nor his mother were known to have had any disqualifying conditions that might have prevented them from owning firearms. In Maryland, a disturbed student took a gun to school and shot another boy in the cafeteria before he was tackled by a teacher; the gun he used was the legal property of his stepfather.

You might ask why a book on involuntary psychiatric care even includes a chapter on firearms. This subject is relevant because crisis-driven laws often come about because we want to do something, even if we don't know what would be best. Legislation to limit gun ownership and to force those with mental illness to get treatment has been promoted as the answer to preventing mass murders, despite the fact that neither common sense nor evidence-based studies support the idea that these measures will prevent these rare atrocities. We discuss these issues in more depth in chapter 21, which specifically looks at mass murderers. While thoughtful gun control legislation might well decrease firearm deaths, the legislation proposed to specifically prevent mass murders does not target the circumstances in which these dangerous individuals have been able to access weapons.

Dan was able to legally obtain a firearm. His pointed question in the gun store didn't dissuade the clerk from selling him a gun, and his unusual and seclusive behavior at work would not be a reason to forbid someone from owning a weapon. Fortunately, he never used his firearm to harm anyone.

What Swanson thinks would be useful is legislation that allows for the preemptive seizure of firearms. Current law in most states is directed at identifying people with mental illness or a history of felony crimes and reporting them to a database. Then, checking to see if they own guns and sending a notice that those guns need to be turned in is a process that takes time. In Maryland, if psychiatrists are concerned that a patient is dangerous, they can send the police to bring the patient to the emergency room for evaluation, where the ED physician may or may not agree to hospitalize the person; they cannot send the police specifically to confiscate a patient's weapons. The officer may only ask the patient to voluntarily give up the weapons. If the person is released from the emergency room, the weapons must be returned.

One solution to this problem is being explored in California. Anyone who has been placed under a restraining order due to domestic violence is required to surrender their weapon to police or to sell the weapon to a licensed dealer within 24 hours of being served with the restraining order. In 2014, following a mass shooting near the University of California's Santa Barbara campus, that law was expanded to allow concerned family members to petition a judge to remove firearms from anyone they feared might be mentally unstable or violent. If granted, the petition allows police to confiscate weapons for up to 21 days, or up to a year if the petition is extended. This is the first law that allows the removal of weapons for reasons other than domestic violence or an overt criminal act. The person who is subject to the order is also barred from purchasing a gun for up to five years following the expiration of the order.

Following his skirmish with the police, Dan was hospitalized on a psychiatric unit briefly, then charged with assault. All told, he spent a number of weeks in the custody of both the mental health system and the criminal justice system. Because his psychosis was seen as a mitigating factor, he was placed on probation before judgment and did not spend more time in jail, but he is no longer able to legally purchase a firearm.

19

Bryan Stanley, Violence, and Psychiatric Illness

Lily's behavior was disruptive, but she was never obviously dangerous to herself or anyone else. She had no history of violence, nor was she threatening to harm anyone. Eleanor also had no history of violence and was not threatening to harm anyone. During her hospitalization, however, the nursing notes referred to her as aggressive and assaultive, without giving explanations.

"I was not the best-behaved patient," Eleanor said.

One day she tried to escape from the unit by blending in with someone else's family as they were leaving after a visit. Another day she pulled the fire alarm with the hope that she could escape during an evacuation. Later, she blockaded herself in her room—and her roommate out of the room—and believed a SWAT team was coming to rescue her. Eleanor became convinced that the cameras on the unit were filming a "mental patient reality TV show," and she went from room to room to warn the other patients. The nursing notes indicated that she dialed 911 and asked the police to come to the unit. On yet another occasion, she threw her arms around a patient in the dayroom, trying to offer an unwanted hug.

While these actions were certainly disruptive and perhaps frightening to other patients, they didn't qualify as violent. As we've mentioned, Eleanor was hospitalized for being gravely disabled, not for being dangerous. When I asked why the chart documented that she was assaultive, all Eleanor could say was that she might have fought back when orderlies held her down to inject medications; she did not recall any episodes of unprovoked violence.

In his book *The Insanity Offense*, Dr. Torrey championed the belief that since people with severe mental illness can be unpredictably violent, they should be involuntarily hospitalized and treated. He wrote of two major "disasters" in mental health care in the United States: deinstitutionalization and the legal profession. Torrey believes that civil rights attorneys have contributed to the creation of laws that prevent very ill people from getting the care they need.

"I have said many times that deinstitutionalization was fundamentally a good idea," Torrey clarified when we spoke. "It became a disaster only *when we failed to provide treatment* for half the patients discharged. Most of these individuals do not need to be hospitalized, but can be involuntarily medicated using assisted outpatient treatment."

In his book, he told story after story of people with mental illnesses who committed heinous crimes. To the general public, some of these crimes might appear predictable, and the stories are formulaic. The patient had a long history of psychosis and violence. Involuntary care provided temporary help, but once the patient was no longer dangerous, he was released from the hospital, only to relapse and become violent again. The stories all have a disastrous ending, often the murder of a family member.

Torrey's accounts, however, do not tell the complete story of the mentally ill person who commits a violent act, nor do they illustrate how courts and mental health professionals struggle to determine which behaviors indicate future violence. We borrow one of Torrey's stories to explain this in more detail.

Bryan Stanley was a veteran and an avid outdoorsman from Wisconsin who developed schizophrenia in the military. He was given a medical discharge and a small pension. After his military service, he was hospitalized and medicated involuntarily a number of times. While Torrey reported that Stanley had a good response to medications, he also noted that Stanley would not take them because he didn't believe he was ill.

According to local newspapers, Stanley was brought to the Emergency Department by police twice for evaluation, only to be released when mental health professionals deemed him safe. Days after the last evaluation, Stanley walked into his church with a shotgun and killed his priest, a lay minister, and the janitor—a particularly brutal crime for a small Wisconsin town. Newspaper reports noted that Stanley believed he was a prophet on a mission to cleanse the church. He had confronted the priest earlier and told him he didn't want "girls" reading the scriptures at mass, and when the priest did not respond favorably, Stanley returned with his gun. At trial, Stanley was found not guilty by reason of insanity and was sent to the Mendota Mental Health Institute for long-term, inpatient treatment.

In the previous chapter, we discussed firearms and mental illness and touched on the issue of mental illness and violence in general. Sorting out the relationship between the two is a complicated task that has confounded psychiatric researchers for years. This isn't too surprising when you consider the ethics and the practical impossibility of doing this research; you can't randomly assign people you think might be dangerous to treatment in the community while giving another set of patients placebo treatments.

Another challenge is that there are many definitions of "violence" in psychiatric research. Shouting, making a verbal threat, or breaking property could all be considered violent behavior, but those actions are not counted as violence in some research studies. Some studies use criminal records to measure violence, but most assaults are never reported to police, especially if they don't lead to injury.

There is also a difference between knowing a risk factor for a problem and using that risk factor to predict a specific event. For example, we know that smoking is a risk factor for heart disease, but we can't predict exactly which smoker will have a heart attack or when exactly that heart attack will happen. There are people who live long, healthy lives even though they smoke while others die earlier from unrelated causes before tobacco has a chance to do them in. Similarly, meteorologists can use satellite data to monitor global storm patterns and seismologists can monitor a global network of earth motion data, but even with this information they can only forecast hurricanes and earthquakes to a certain degree of probability and for a limited time into the future. Catastrophic events are impossible to predict exactly, and the prediction problem is magnified for events that are extremely rare, like violence committed by psychiatric patients. Surely, if the doctors who saw Stanley in the Emergency Department knew that he would kill people, they would have kept him. In fact, as Dr. Skivorski pointed out in the chapter on emergency psychiatry, the ED doctors likely would have kept Stanley if they believed there was even a small risk that he'd kill people.

The first large-scale study to consider violence by psychiatric patients used data gathered during the National Institute of Mental Health's Epidemiologic Catchment Area study in the early 1980s. Researchers interviewed 10,024 randomly chosen people in Baltimore, Raleigh-Durham, and Los Angeles. They asked questions about past psychiatric diagnoses, treatment, and substance use. They asked about any acts of violence the people had committed in the year prior to the interview, as well as the history of violence over the person's lifetime. Interviewers found that 90 percent of the people with mental illness reported they had never been violent. The self-reported one-year prevalence of violence among people with mental illness was about 7 percent.

Having any psychiatric diagnosis, particularly a diagnosis of schizophrenia, did increase the risk of violence. People who had more than one psychiatric diagnosis had a risk of violence that rose in proportion to the number of psychiatric diagnoses. The combination of substance abuse and major psychopathology was particularly predictive; nearly one-third of those diagnosed with both schizophrenia and substance abuse had been violent. However, certain nonclinical factors were also significant predictors of violence: being young, male, and having a lower socioeconomic status.

A national survey published in 2012 found remarkably similar results. People with both serious mental illness and substance abuse problems had the highest rate of violence: nearly three times the rate of people with mental illness who didn't abuse drugs or alcohol. These researchers also found that people who suffered abuse or neglect in childhood and those raised by parents with criminal involvement or drug and alcohol abuse were at risk for behaving violently even in the absence of mental illness. Stressful life events were also associated with violence in the absence of mental illness. In this study, receiving mental health care in the community did not reduce the risk of violence, but there were too few people in treatment to rule out the utility of clinical intervention. Out of 34,000 people who were surveyed, only 12.8 percent were in treatment.

There were other associations as well, which violence researcher Dr. Jeffrey Swanson pointed out when we discussed guns and mental illness—poverty, substance abuse, and previous exposure to violence.

"If you take away all those factors and just look at people with serious mental illness, then the rates of violence are about 2 percent in a year, the same as in the general population without mental illness. But once you start adding those factors, then violence increases."

Swanson talked about a University of Pittsburgh study that followed patients discharged from an emergency room and compared their rates of violence against the predictions of two psychiatrists. Just over half of the patients who were predicted to be violent did commit a violent act. But 36 percent of those deemed to be not violent committed an act of violence. With female patients, the psychiatrists did no better than chance.

In his book, Torrey contended that if we kept people with chronic psychiatric disorders in treatment, violent crimes would not happen. Most people would agree in retrospect, and the story of Bryan Stanley certainly argues for more use of involuntary, longer-term care. But emergency room clinicians and courts don't have the luxury of hindsight when they make decisions about detaining people. As a society, we've decided that it is wrong to hold people *forever* at a facility against their will because they *might* commit a crime in the future, and the courts' interpretation of the US Constitution requires each state to periodically review the need to keep someone institutionalized. Even if Stanley had been hospitalized involuntarily after one of his emergency room visits, the law required that the doctors release him as soon as he was safe for discharge. And as we have repeatedly seen, merely being delusional is not a strong indicator of future dangerousness.

"I can understand why some people would disagree and say that no one should ever be treated involuntarily unless they've demonstrated dangerousness," Torrey said when I met with him.

But if you take that position, then you also have to accept the number of homeless mentally ill we have now. And you have to accept most of the ones that are in jail and prison: there are 10 times more people with mental illness in the jails and prisons than there are in the remaining state hospital beds. And you also have to accept a certain number of homicides. I have stated, and I think the data support it, that about 10 percent of homicides are committed by people with untreated, severe mental illness, which is about 1,300 homicides a year. So I understand why people would argue that nobody should ever be treated involuntarily, but I would also argue then that you have to accept the consequences, because it does have consequences.

Forensic psychiatrist Paul Appelbaum talked about how involuntary treatment might impact the rates of violent crime. His views differed from Torrey's.

Violence driven by delusions clearly happens. There's conflicting literature on whether the presence of delusions increases violence overall. It's clear that merely having a delusion does not. But there is evidence that if you're delusional, and angry as a result, then you are at higher risk for violence than you are without anger, even if the same kind of persecutory delusion is present. That being said, there are several studies that suggest that most violence by persons with serious mental illness doesn't relate to their serious mental illness.

Overall, the amount of violence attributable to mental illness in the United States is about 4 percent, so that's the ceiling for the effect that you can have with all mentally ill people. Now we're talking about a very small group of people with untreated, early phase mental illness, and just about a very particular kind, so the impact is going to be tiny. The rates of serious violence are sufficiently low that you'd end up committing 50 people or more for every act of violence that you were looking to prevent. It wouldn't be a very good way of going about doing it.

The most ambitious and most often cited study of violence and mental illness is the MacArthur Violence Risk Assessment Study. Researchers followed 951 recently discharged psychiatric inpatients for one year and compared self-reported violent acts with medical and legal records and with information from collateral informants, such as friends and relatives. Of the patients available for at least one follow-up, 262 (28 percent) committed at least one act of violence. A total of 608 violent acts were committed by these 262 patients. In the absence of substance abuse, patients with mental illness were no more violent than other people in the same community. For those who were violent, the victim was most often a family member and the violence took place at home.

The MacArthur violence study found that most recently discharged patients were not violent. The risk of violence was higher for men, for people with previous histories of violent behavior, for people with traumatic or abusive childhoods, and for people who came from minority or economically disadvantaged communities. Certain personality characteristics were also relevant. People with psychopathic traits, those who admitted to having violent thoughts, and those who had high levels of anger were more likely to commit violent acts.

A critic of the MacArthur study, Torrey pointed out that of the 951 discharged patients followed in the study, three of them killed six people. He noted that one patient had been talking to the television and otherwise behaving strangely, and may have been delusional when he killed his girlfriend. A second patient had been hearing multiple voices and may also have been delusional before he killed someone. Since the identities of these patients are unknown, we have no way of determining if they were declared legally insane once the evidence was presented at trial or if the crimes were completely independent of their illnesses.

An in-depth review published in 2008 of the MacArthur study attempted to clarify the relationship, if any, between psychotic symptoms and patients' violent behavior. The researchers identified all the discharged patients who were involved in two or more incidents of violence during the year after hospital discharge. They found that 100 repeatedly violent patients accounted for half of the violent incidents. They reviewed the responses to the original interview questions about the patients' thoughts immediately prior to the incidents and about the presence of hallucinations. Then they classified each violent patient into one of three categories: patients who had violence exclusively preceded by psychotic symptoms, those whose violence never followed psychotic symptoms, and those whose violence was inconsistently preceded by psychosis.

Psychotic symptoms preceded the violence in only 12 percent of the 305 incidents reviewed. Eighty percent of the repeatedly violent patients did not experience psychotic symptoms before any of their violent incidents. The authors concluded that "effective treatment of psychosis will have negligible direct effects on violence for most patients and important but partial effects for the remainder." In other words, an intervention that only addresses mental illness is unlikely to be effective in preventing the violence of repeatedly violent patients.

Another study incidentally helped tease out the relationship between psychotic symptoms and violence, although the primary purpose was to look at the cost efficacy of new antipsychotic medications. Researchers sponsored by the National Institute of Mental Health interviewed 1,410 patients with schizophrenia and asked about violent behavior in the preceding six months. The self-reports were compared with information obtained from family members about each person. Eighty percent of the patients were never violent, and only 3.6 percent had an incident of serious violence, such as an assault that resulted in injury. Patients with the negative symptoms of schizophrenia, including social withdrawal and apathy, were at less risk of violence than patients without these symptoms. Another protective factor was a supportive family environment. Patients who felt listened to by their family members were half as likely to behave violently as subjects who did not feel listened to by family.

Family relationships are important; family members can reduce the risk of violence, but they are also most likely to be the victim of a violent mentally ill person. Treating psychotic symptoms may help in specific cases, but treatment is less likely to help if the person has underlying impulse control problems or an irritable temperament, issues similar to those that we discussed in the chapter on guns and mental illness. One of the more interesting findings of the MacArthur study, to us, was that being delusional generally did not make someone more violent, but being angry about the delusion did.

John Monahan, a psychologist and professor at the University of Virginia School of Law, studies the prediction of violent behavior. In a symposium on dangerousness and involuntary mental health treatment held at the University of Pennsylvania in March 2014 Monahan said, "Reluctantly, the bottom line is that there is some relationship between mental illness and violence. Advocates deny this and say the rate is the same, but it's not the case that there is *no* relationship."

Monahan reiterated what Swanson said when discussing mental illness and gun violence: it's not simply an issue of mental illness. Substance abuse is a much stronger predictor of violence, and the combination of substance abuse, mental illness, and exposure to community violence dramatically increases the chance that any given person will be violent.

Monahan discussed how *voluntary* treatment can mitigate this risk. "People in weekly treatment were less violent than the general population," he noted. It's an interesting point, given how rare it is for voluntary patients treated at community mental health centers to be offered weekly visits.

We are left with the question of whether involuntary care prevents violence, and this is something we just don't know. Holding people in a hospital certainly decreases the likelihood that they will present a danger to the general public. There are patients who elope (or escape) from the hospital, and as we mentioned in chapter 12, there are certainly instances of violence—including murders and suicides—that occur inside a psychiatric unit. Overall, it seems that if someone is acutely and imminently dangerous to others—with or without a mental illness diagnosis—then institutionalization in some type of facility would decrease risk.

But how long should an admission continue in order to ensure that a person is safe to release? And what steps should society take to be certain that people who are both dangerous and mentally ill receive care in the community if they are refusing voluntary treatment—or if they have a history of agreeing to such treatment, but then don't comply? If the goal is violence prevention, how do we make certain that we only involuntarily hold those people who actually will be violent and not scores of others, given that psychiatrists don't have crystal balls and that involuntary treatment is distressing to many people?

And what happened to Bryan Stanley?

Stanley was hospitalized at a state forensic facility for 23 years. During that time he was prescribed an antipsychotic medication, fluphenazine. He took the medication voluntarily and regularly, until he began to refuse the medication because he said it caused sedation, tremors, pain in his feet and lower legs, and restlessness. The medication was changed to a different one, clozapine, and on the new medication, he had a remarkable recovery. He was able to move to a minimum security unit within the hospital and ultimately was allowed to leave the hospital grounds, unescorted, to take computer courses at a local college. He was able to travel by city bus to a part-time job and to take a correspondence course through a local library. He had overnight visits with his family, and he complied with unannounced staff visits and the required telephone check-ins. He even spent six years writing a book, *The Becoming of Driftless Rivers National Park* (2006), to promote interest in preserving the natural resources of southwestern Wisconsin, where he had once spent time fishing, camping, and hunting. He petitioned for conditional release on multiple occasions but was denied by the circuit court each time.

Stanley's treating psychiatrist, an independent court-appointed psychiatrist, and Stanley's case manager all agreed that he was ready for release from the hospital. They testified that he was consistently adherent with his prescribed treatment. They testified about multiple safeguards in place to monitor his mental state and his activities.

By Wisconsin law, the state was required to prove, by clear and convincing evidence, that Stanley posed a significant risk of danger if released from the hospital. In spite of the fact that the state presented no witnesses or documents to make its case, the judge refused release, stating, "Where I may be willing to take the risk had his crime not been what it was, based upon his current treatment plan, I am not willing to take that risk based upon what this crime was all about." In other words, the evidence of Stanley's dangerousness was his crime, and the court disregarded Stanley's 23 years of treatment.

Stanley appealed this decision, and a year later he was granted release by the Wisconsin Court of Appeals. The release sparked concern from the community, from law enforcement, and from the media. The *La-Crosse Tribune* sued the court system to get Stanley's new address. He had moved into a small home purchased by a corporation owned by his brother. In a story published by the local newspaper, his neighbors described him as "quiet and friendly."

After three years in the community, Stanley's conditional release was revoked, and he was sent back to the hospital not because of violent behavior, not because of a refusal to comply with treatment, and not because of a new crime, but because he was having violent thoughts. Stanley had told a nurse at a VA facility about these thoughts. This was then reported to his case manager and his probation agent. He was rehospitalized, and later investigation revealed that he had been having violent thoughts toward women for the previous two years. Some of those thoughts were focused on a woman he had lent money to and a family member. He had finally told the nurse about the thoughts because they bothered him, and he did not want to act on them; he wanted help.

The court revoked his conditional release, asserting that it was a violation of the release conditions because he had not reported his intrusive violent thoughts to his psychiatrist sooner. As of this writing, Bryan Stanley remains in a state facility for the ongoing treatment of his schizophrenia.

Most people would find it hard to fault a judge for rehospitalizing someone who had killed three people and who was having violent thoughts again, or for making a hospital discharge difficult for someone with this history of violence. In this case, it might be even more understandable because Stanley's initial crime occurred soon after two Emergency Departments had released him; his crime was not predictable. But when it comes to preventing serious violence, we have to consider the fact that having *any* psychiatric diagnosis raises the risk of violence just slightly. Presently there aren't enough psychiatric hospital beds to admit even people who are symptomatic, including those seeking treatment on a voluntary basis. And as the Stanley case illustrates, once you get committed to a hospital, it can be awfully hard to get out.

20

Amy and Involuntary Treatment for Suicide Prevention

For most of this book, we've focused on patients who suffer from psychotic disorders—illnesses characterized by hallucinations, delusions, and disorganized thinking. Proponents of involuntary care often stress that some of these patients are not even aware they have a mental illness; they refuse to get treatment because they see it as unnecessary, if not intrusive. The illness, the proponents of involuntary care contend, robs the patient of the capacity to make a choice in much the same way that Alzheimer's disease might.

Many patients, however, are hospitalized because they are at risk of suicide rather than in need of treatment for psychosis. Suicide in the United States is a public health crisis: the rates have been steadily increasing since 2000, and more than 40,000 people took their own lives in 2013. It is currently the tenth leading cause of death overall, and the third leading cause of death in the 15–24 age group. While much of the outcry about involuntary treatment is about mass murderers, the attention they get in terms of funding and legislation for mental health problems is disproportionate to the rarity of those crimes.

Most—if not the vast majority—of the people who die of suicide are believed to be suffering from a mental illness. Many have a mood disorder, such as major depression or bipolar disorder, but suicide rates are also notably elevated in people with schizophrenia and other psychiatric conditions. One estimate is that 90 percent of suicide deaths occur in people who have psychiatric disorders, both treated and untreated.

Suicide is often an impulsive event, and suicide rates can be reduced by limiting access to lethal methods. According to the Centers for Disease Control, guns are one of the most common means of suicide, second only to hanging. According to one national survey, having a gun in the home triples the risk of homicide and increases the risk of suicide more than twenty times. While we can't control access to ropes and we can't keep people off bridges, communities have tried to intervene by posting signs on bridges with a suicide hotline number and by placing safety barriers on bridges to prevent fatal falls or jumps. Suicidal people are often ambivalent about death, so offering an opportunity to talk to someone about it or placing an obstacle that delays the action can be life-saving.

A close brush with a near-lethal attempt can also change someone's mind about wanting to die. Jumping from the Golden Gate Bridge is nearly always fatal, but some people have survived the jump into the frigid waters of San Francisco Bay. A follow-up study of a group of survivors showed that only 6 percent went on to die of suicide.

While not all suicides are impulsive or even preventable, a brief hospitalization may keep people safe long enough to get them through a bad moment in life. Treatment can be offered for depression, which eases suffering. A nonjudgmental and supportive outpatient clinician can help a distressed person solve a problem or can provide needed social support.

Although emergency room clinicians are trained to assess suicide risk and to weigh protective factors against suicide risk factors, ultimately only patients know the seriousness of their intent. Stated suicidal intent, or denial of intent, is considered along with other information gathered during the evaluation. Sometimes the decision to admit or discharge suicidal patients is made based on their actions. For example, a "farewell" post on social media by a teenager may be read as having ominous meaning, but if the teen insists she is safe and family members confirm that she was happily planning a future social event earlier in the day, she might be released. In contrast, doctors are often hesitant to release a person after a self-inflicted injury. A patient's ardent reassurance, however, can be quite convincing, and it is not unheard of for a person to be released from an ED or discharged from a psychiatric unit and then die of suicide hours later.

There are no psychological scales or scientific algorithms to follow that will guarantee a successful outcome, and much of a physician's decision making is intuition. Logistical issues may also play a role, including whether beds are available, whether outpatient resources are available, and the patient's stated willingness and ability to continue treatment after release from the emergency room. A patient who has family support and a psychiatrist who will see her the next morning is less likely to be involuntarily hospitalized than one who would be sent home alone with no reasonable prospect of getting an appointment anytime soon. Financial factors also come into play when it comes to obtaining a bed for any patient.

Because many of the stories in this book are told from the vantage point of those who felt injured by involuntary care, for this chapter we purposely recruited patients who felt helped by their treatment.

Amy (not her real name) grew up in a wonderful family and had a happy childhood. However, her life abruptly changed when she was 11: her older brother died in a car accident. "He was my hero. He would bring ice cream into my class and volunteer to help. I didn't realize how unusual that was for a big brother. When he died, I tried to pretend it didn't happen, but the next year, I had my first suicide attempt, and I truly wanted and expected to die."

As if there wasn't already enough tragedy in this family, Amy's father died when she was 13. She described a tumultuous adolescence, and she spent several months in a psychiatric hospital during her junior year of high school. Still, Amy did well in school and was given a full scholarship to attend college. Leaving home, however, did not go smoothly. Amy was hospitalized for a few days during the fall of her freshman year for cutting herself. The rest of the year did not go any better.

"There was a time when I actually tried to go to the hospital myself, when I felt horribly suicidal. I told the psychiatrist I was feeling suicidal, and he responded, 'What do you want me to do, tie your hands behind your back?' I went home and that night took 80 or so antidepressants and ended up in the ICU, and then in a psych ward."

At the end of the year, the college told Amy not to return. "I was deeply hurt. But they had tried to meet with me and create a plan, and I was too sick to be there. I was getting straight A's, but I could have easily killed myself, and I was very depressed and wanted to die. It ended up being the best thing for me not to return."

Amy moved home and went to a local university, and things started to go better. Over the course of several years, she graduated from college, married, had her first child, and worked at several interesting jobs.

"I don't know why I was okay for those five years. It was a respite from being mentally ill. But I became depressed again, and it was like someone reached in with one of those claws in those amusement machines and lifted me out of my life and dropped me on a crazy train!"

She recounted a nightmarish cycle of pain, self-harm, asking for help, and hospitalizations. Amy told stories of cutting herself and then going to an urgent care center for stitches, of overdosing in her car and then asking a stranger to call the police. In one instance, she cut herself while she was in the emergency room with a razor blade she had hidden behind her cell phone battery. In another, she overdosed on Xanax while in a seclusion room.

Amy noted that during one admission the doctors wanted to send her to a state hospital. Her family was against it, and she called a lawyer. The hearing was held in a public courtroom, and her family asked to have everyone leave, for which Amy was grateful. She didn't want her problems announced in open court. The judge released her at the hearing. Amy said, "I won the hearing, but I wasn't okay. I went to counseling three days a week, and I went back to work. But I was still brutally depressed."

After yet another suicide attempt, Amy was taken to a hospital in an adjacent state. "I liked my doctors there—they were kind—but I didn't feel better, and I decided I would kill myself."

After Amy was discharged, she left the hospital alone and tried to kill herself again. This time, she ended up in a state hospital and began getting specialized behavioral therapy to help her cope better with her emotions. Known as dialectical behavioral therapy, this is the same treatment that helped Marsha, the patient on court-ordered outpatient care. "This time, my only job was to work on me, and I finally became convinced that wellness was possible for me."

Eventually, things improved. Amy stopped feeling excruciating psychic pain and stopped trying to hurt herself, and since then she has remained out of the hospital and off medications. She and her husband have had two more children, and she has returned to school to get a graduate degree. She gives her family—particularly her husband—and friends credit for helping her get through such difficult times.

"What I've told you about is my periods of craziness. This doesn't include all the joys, which outnumber the tears by a thousandfold."

Amy's story had so many different turns, events, and hospitalizations that it was hard to keep track of the details. In some instances, she didn't know if her hospitalizations were voluntary or not. Suicidal patients are often told that they need to come into the hospital in much the same way that someone is admitted for a heart attack or pneumonia. Patients may sign in and not realize they had a choice, and they might assume they were there on an involuntary basis. Involuntarily admitted suicidal patients are often discharged in a matter of days, before a formal commitment hearing is held. Amy said that only one of her hospitalizations felt voluntary, and since she does recall having a court hearing, it seems she could not simply sign herself out for at least one of her admissions.

Did hospitalization save Amy? I asked.

"The hospital kept my medications locked up, which kept me from acting on my suicidal impulses. It would have been better if they also spent more time providing positive ways to cope when my feelings were very intense. I walked the halls quite a bit and colored and listened to music. This was helpful. The lack of personal autonomy and isolation from family and friends were not."

Amy talked about her recent successes and all the wonderful people in her life with wistfulness. "This is what I would have missed if I had killed myself. As crazy as it is to hear, it was even crazier living it."

Sherry (not her real name) wrote in with her thoughts on her involuntary hospitalization:

Ironically, although the hospitalization was involuntary and I was so torn up about going, it was one of the most useful experiences I've had since my introduction to psychiatry, perhaps as much as medication. First off, I was safe from myself when my mind was going haywire, and I had a good reason to be excused from school and responsibilities and from trying to pretend everything was okay in front of my friends, which was an enormous relief. Secondly, I was in the ward with a wonderful group of people. They all had serious struggles, but they were charming and calm and friendly and fun. It didn't make crazy seem so crazy. We all really opened up to each other, and while I was only there four days, it was massively supportive and caring and generous and structured and peaceful and safe. Thirdly, there were a host of mental health care professionals on tap, all the time. I was almost sorry to go when I was discharged. Almost. Having a real bed, access to my phone, regular showers, and the ability to shave again was fantastic.

Amy's and Sherry's stories demonstrate the challenge of assessing suicide risk and the importance of short-term involuntary admissions. Amy's behaviors and stated intentions all confirmed that she was a danger to herself, while Sherry talked about her ability to "pretend everything was okay in front of my friends." Doctors have to decide if patients are pretending to be well, and they have to intervene when someone self-injures, even if the patient's intent may not be death. Doctors are afraid of making a fatal mistake. The tendency remains to hospitalize suicidal people when there is doubt, with a "better safe than sorry" outlook. Even if we concede that involuntary hospitalization may be traumatizing, many would contend that it's better to have many traumatized patients than a single dead patient.

How often is civil commitment used for patients with suicidal risk as compared to patients with psychosis? There are no statistics on such things. It may well depend on who is in the Emergency Department. As we saw in the chapter on emergency rooms, psychiatrists may be more comfortable than ED physicians in releasing people at risk for suicide, and both psychiatrists and ED doctors may be less likely to discharge someone who is actively psychotic.

Dr. Robert Roca, the vice president and medical director of Sheppard Pratt Health System in Baltimore, said, "We don't have data readily at hand that answer that question. It's fair to say that the vast majority of patients admitted because of suicidality come in voluntarily. Many, if not most, involuntary patients admitted for this reason are transferred from EDs or a medical-surgical hospital following actual suicide attempts."

It's likely that many of the voluntary patients felt coerced. Some may have been told that if they didn't sign in, they would be admitted against their will.

When asked about the involuntary treatment of people who are suicidal but not psychotic, Dr. Torrey stated that he had no expertise with this patient population. "Suicide can be, and often is, a fully rational decision," he said. "I won't say I would never involuntarily hospitalize such a person, but it would take a very unusual set of circumstances."

Robert Bossarte, PhD, is an epidemiologist who studies suicide for the Veterans Administration.

"We are looking at people who were hospitalized after their first suicide attempt and looking at rates of mortality and suicidal behavior for one year after discharge," he said. "It's preliminary evidence, but we didn't see any difference in the outcome. If a person is hospitalized for a first suicide attempt, and we followed them for a year and focused on all-cause mortality or repeat suicide attempts, we were not able to identify a difference between those who were hospitalized and those who were not. We don't yet know about completed suicides."

Designing a study to answer this question is a challenge because, like studying violence by psychiatric patients, there is no way to ethically do a randomized controlled trial of treatment for suicidal patients. However, we do have evidence that mental health services can reduce suicide deaths. This evidence comes from an unexpected source, American jails and prisons.

In 1972 inmate David Ruiz sued the Texas Department of Corrections over a wide range of inhumane living conditions and a lack of services in that state's prison system. His suit became one of the most famous class action cases in the history of correctional litigation and marked the beginning of several decades of prison reform. Among his allegations was a complaint about the lack of mental health services and inadequate medical care. The federal district court agreed and established a list of mental health services that the prison system should provide. This list is now considered a national standard, which every facility must meet in order to provide constitutionally adequate care.

Each correctional facility must have a system to screen and identify inmates in need of mental health services, including those at risk of suicide, and it must have adequate numbers of trained mental health professionals to provide care. Each jail and prison must also have a suicide prevention program.

After the *Ruiz* decision, the rate of inmate suicide deaths dropped dramatically. Between 1983 and 1999, the suicide rate in US jails dropped to 54 per 100,000 from 129 per 100,000. The suicide rate in prisons decreased to 15 per 100,000 from 27 per 100,000 over the same time period. This reduction is particularly impressive, given that many inmates have at least three risk factors for suicide: being young, being male, and having an active substance abuse problem. The additional stresses of a criminal prosecution and a harsh correctional environment don't help either. But when treatment is available, and efforts are made to reach out to those who need it, lives can be saved.

There are those who believe that people should have the right to end their own lives and that suicidal people, even those with a psychiatric disorder, should not be committed to hospitals against their will. Psychiatrists generally believe otherwise: suicide may be an impulsive act, and keeping someone safe for a short period may be enough to save a life. Furthermore, the distinction between dangerousness to self and dangerousness to others may not be black and white. One suicidal pilot purposely crashed a commercial airliner, killing hundreds of people on board. Severely depressed mothers have killed their children. The Sandy Hook, Virginia Tech, and Columbine killers all died as part of their planned acts of violence. And sometimes people unintentionally harm others during violent acts intended to harm only themselves.

We justify involuntary care because suicidal thoughts are often part of a treatable psychiatric illness. Suicide is rarely a benign ending; the families and friends left behind are devastated. And we aggressively try to prevent suicide because we hate to see people die when there may still be the promise of a joyful and productive life, just as Amy described.

Will Forcing Treatment on People with Psychiatric Disorders Prevent Mass Murders?

We started this book with the idea that involuntary psychiatric treatment has been proposed as a possible solution to mass murders. We have specifically mentioned the graduate student in Aurora who killed people in a crowded movie theater, the Tucson gunman who killed six people and shot a US representative at a political rally, and the man in Newtown who killed 27 people in an elementary school. We will never know all the facts of these crimes.

The Tucson shooter pled guilty, so a trial was never held, and the evidence was never presented. The Newtown shooter committed suicide, so we will never know what thoughts and feelings led to such an atrocity. The Aurora movie theater shooter entered an insanity plea, but was found guilty of his crime and sentenced to life in prison without the possiblity of parole. Without an evaluation or access to investigation records, we will not speculate on the role mental illness may have played in these crimes. Here, we present the opinions of others and the results of investigations where they are available to highlight the problems surrounding the use of involuntary treatment to prevent these crimes.

There are people who believe that mass murders can be prevented through legislation. After the massacre at Newtown, Representative Timothy Murphy wrote in the *Guardian*:

> I remain firmly convinced we can make tremendous legislative strides in preventing mass tragedies involving someone with a serious mental illness. And just as importantly, we can save countless lives of those with

mental illness from suicide, victimization, homelessness and despair. We owe it to the Newtown families to take meaningful action—to fix the chaotic patchwork of programs and laws that make it impossible to get meaningful medical care until it is too late to [do] anything beyond mourning. To do nothing is a shame on us all, and a disservice to the Sandy Hook victims and parents who courageously face each day in the midst of their pain. Let their courage be our motivation to take action—now.

Dr. E. Fuller Torrey agreed that these shooting sprees were caused by failures of the mental health system:

I have a pretty good guess of what happened to [the shooter in Tucson], which is that three months prior to his "evaluation" when he was kicked out of college, the state legislature had gutted the funds for the program of involuntary treatment—and I really mean gutted in terms of the money—and the word then came down to Pima County saying they needed to cut down on this very expensive involuntary treatment because it's very expensive. So the local community mental health center, of [which] the chief of police for the Pima Community College was on the board—so she was very aware of this—they were aware that the last thing the Pima Community Mental Health Center wanted was for them to bring him down and hospitalize him. I strongly suspect that played a role in their final decision. In addition, the lawyers from the college would have said, "Inform his parents and then we're out of here," because that's what lawyers do. So I think the decision was made, not based on his needs but based on the fact that the program he would have been treated under had been financially gutted, and because the lawyers will always opt to do as little as possible so that nobody will sue them.

Torrey went on to discuss the financial issues he thought may have played a role in keeping another mass murderer from getting care. "With the fellow in Colorado, clearly there were red flags all over the place. I have a pretty good guess. The inpatient unit had been closed down the year before, the one I think he would have gone to. So the availability of beds to hospitalize him were limited, and again, I suspect the university lawyers played a role and advised them to do as little as possible."

As we discussed in chapter 19, violence by a person with mental illness is not common. Although also an extremely rare event, mass murder has been happening with increasing frequency in the twenty-first century. In order to shape a national emergency management policy to respond to these incidents, the Congressional Research Service produced the report *Public Mass Shootings in the United States: Selected Implications for Federal Public Health and Safety Policy* in March 2013. This report summarized certain statistics related to mass shooting events. It recorded 78 mass shootings from 1983 to the time of the report, resulting in 547 deaths and 476 injuries.

An exhaustive look at mass shooting incidents was published in *Mother Jones*, and the magazine updates the data with every new tragedy. As of December 2015, it had recorded 73 such attacks. The Congressional Research Service report relied in part on the database developed by these journalists, so it's not surprising the results are similar. The *Mother Jones* story reported 69 mass murders in the United States from 1982 to 2012. Sixty-eight of the shooters were men; only one was a woman. Most bought their guns legally, and some exhibited symptoms of mental illness, though many of them had not come to the attention of mental health professionals. Thirty-six of the gunmen died by suicide at the scene of the shooting; seven more were killed by the police.

Both the congressional report and the *Mother Jones* story defined a "mass murder" as an incident in which four or more victims are killed, excluding the shooter, in a relatively public place. Both the report and the story excluded crimes in which the motive was robbery or terrorism, as well as cases of domestic violence. This definition is clearly restrictive, since a mass shooting at a public workplace could be motivated by domestic violence and so would be excluded. The requirement that the murders take place at a public location leaves out family annihilation crimes, in which an individual kills his entire family in a private home. Similarly, gang and drug-related shootings are excluded. And finally, the number of "mass shootings," where four or more people are wounded without that many deaths, is much greater than the number of mass murders. The numbers presented in these reports are therefore likely to be underestimates.

The mass murderers of strangers in public places are singled out because it is assumed that their psychological makeup and motivations are different from the psychological makeup and motivations of people who kill those they know. Although the gunman who is tackled after shooting one or two strangers would not meet the definition of a mass murderer, he might well share some of the characteristics of those whose crimes claim more victims.

We focus on mass murders because these are what the media and the public focus on, and these crimes against innocent strangers in public settings are more likely to be attributed to mental illness, to inspire fear, and to guide discussions of legislation. They are, however, only a small slice of the overall gun violence in the United States.

Regardless of the definition used, and in spite of how common these tragedies are in media reports, we want to put these numbers into perspective. According to the *Mother Jones* data, 2012 was the deadliest year for mass murders, with seven events. That same year, the US population was nearly 313 million. The probability that any given person would be a mass murderer was less than one in 44 million. In 2014, there were two mass murders, and the population had grown to 317 million. The probability of any randomly chosen person being a mass murderer was only one in 158 million. When it comes to being killed by a mass shooter, the odds are equally improbable. According to the Centers for Disease Control, more people are killed every year by dogs, cows, and even bees.

Criminologists have put a lot of effort into methods to classify and identify killers before they act. They have created typologies based on psychiatric diagnosis, motive, type of weapon used, and the killer's relationship with the victim or victims. They have tried to identify characteristics that distinguish school shooters from other mass murderers, and adolescent shooters from adults. The diversity of spree shooters can be seen in the wide variety of settings where mass murder takes place: businesses, shopping malls, schools and universities, government offices, restaurants, parking lots, health-care facilities, and churches. The variety of crime scenes tells us a lot about motivation, which in turn illustrates the challenge of preventing these incidents.

Shopping malls, for example, are targeted by killers looking for a rapid law enforcement response with the maximum potential for publicity and a high body count. Churches may indicate a racial, religious, or ethnic motivation for the crime or may be chosen by a psychotic person with a religious delusion.

The idea that there is one prototypical mass murderer with easily identifiable characteristics is a myth. In the words of the congressional report, "No effective mass shooter profile exists for law enforcement to use to proactively identify potential suspects. . . . Aside from usually but not always being male, there are few other characteristics across mass murderers that would be reliable or valid for creating a general profile for individuals most likely to engage in a public mass shooting." You can use a magnet to look for a needle in a haystack, but we have no tool to pick out that one shooter in 158 million people.

While there is no predictive profile, two descriptive studies of mass murderers did identify some common features. In a paper by Hempel and colleagues in 1999 and another by Meloy and colleagues in 2004, the killers were described as socially isolated, chronically angry, and resentful individuals who suffered a sudden major stressor, usually the loss of a relationship or a problem related to employment. While most did not directly threaten their victims prior to the attack, they fantasized and practiced the assault, and even posed for pictures with weapons in hand. Half had at least one psychiatric hospitalization or one visit with a mental health professional prior to the murders. Forty percent were thought to have psychotic symptoms at the time of the murders, usually paranoid or persecutory delusions, and the majority of these also had preexisting personality pathology. Thirty percent, however, had no psychiatric history.

Based on these studies, any preventive policy that only targets people with known mental illness will miss people at risk. On the other hand, even if we limit the presumed population of potential mass murderers to those with serious and persistent mental illnesses with psychotic symptoms, such as schizophrenia and bipolar disorder, this would encompass more than 14 million Americans, an impossible number to watch for. Further, a screen that looked for only severe mental illness would miss those killers who were seen for obsessive compulsive disorder, anxiety disorder, depression, or adjustment disorder. And all methods that tried to identify would-be mass murderers based on mental illness would miss the killers with no psychiatric disorder—a significant number.

Proponents of involuntary care suggest that aggressive mandatory treatment might have prevented the Aurora and Newtown tragedies. According to publicly available information, both perpetrators had already been involved in care voluntarily. The Newtown shooter had been evaluated for anxiety and for developmental delays, particularly with regard to expressive language and social interactions. He reportedly was seen by the Yale child guidance team for an evaluation, in an Emergency Department at Danbury Hospital for anxiety, and by a psychiatrist in the community approximately 20 times. He carried diagnoses of Asperger's (a variant of autism), obsessive compulsive disorder, anxiety, and anorexia, but there was no mention of a psychotic disorder, and the report of the Office of the Child Advocate stated, "After an exhaustive review of records, emails, and conclusions drawn by law enforcement agencies, [the shooter] was not obviously psychotic in the time period leading up to the Sandy Hook Elementary School shooting though he had a history of depression and suicidal ideation that can be seen in his emails during 2011 and 2012."

Similarly, the Aurora shooter was receiving care from his student mental health center. At his trial, his university psychiatrist testified that the gunman said little in therapy and was "socially anxious." The social worker who referred the shooter to psychiatric care described him as one of the most anxious people she had ever seen, and she suspected he suffered from obsessive compulsive disorder. Both professionals were aware of his violent thoughts, but because he never spoke of a plan to harm people and had no identifiable target or victims, he did not meet the criteria for involuntary hospitalization. He withheld the fact that he was compiling an arsenal of weapons and researching locations for a mass murder. Legislation does not have a means to deal with people who lie about their intentions. Most killers do not threaten a specific victim.

Of the potential killers with no prior mental health contacts (for example, chronically angry or resentful people who experience a sudden major loss), some might seek voluntary care if it were available. Treatment reduces, but does not eliminate, the risk of violence in general. It's likely that treatment averts an unknown number of violent crimes, but we have no statistics on the number of crimes that do not occur. It's also possible that some potential killers might be deterred from seeking treatment for fear of being committed to a hospital, mandated to take medications, losing their right to own guns, or a negative impact on their careers. The stigma of a mental health diagnosis remains strong. There is no research that specifically suggests that treatment can lower the risk of spree shootings.

This leaves us with a pool of potentially violent individuals who may signal their intentions but are unwilling to participate in voluntary care. All states have laws to civilly commit people with mental illness to inpatient treatment under these circumstances. However, a short-term involuntary hospitalization will not fundamentally alter an individual's personality, and there would need to be some assurance of long-term follow-up. If involuntary outpatient care is to be considered, there must be services available and a means to enforce compliance with those services. As we discussed in the chapters on outpatient commitment (part 5 of this book), patients can and do abscond from treatment, and there is no consensus on how best to address patients who don't comply with outpatient treatment orders. In fact, this is exactly what happened with the Virginia Tech shooter; he was involuntarily hospitalized briefly, then released from the hospital on a community treatment order. He never went for follow-up care.

Even if there were procedures in place to pick up an absconder, the detention would not happen immediately. In 2015, the state police in Maryland served 9,092 arrest warrants, most for violent criminals and sex offenders. Police would likely balk if they were required to track down and detain people merely for failing to keep a psychiatric appointment.

We have listed these difficulties to highlight why expanding laws to mandate involuntary care will not prevent large-scale tragedies. These events are too rare to be foreseeable, there are too many people who meet the descriptions of would-be mass murderers, and psychiatric disorder is only one piece of a complex puzzle.

Representative Tim Murphy first proposed the Helping Families in Mental Health Crisis Act in 2013 as sweeping legislation to fix the broken mental health system in the United States in response to the Newtown shootings; it was a promise he made to the families of the children who were killed that day. The original legislation would have required all states to adopt outpatient civil commitment laws or risk the loss of federal funding. This component of the bill was so controversial that Representative Ron Barber (D) of Arizona (one of the victims of the Tucson shooter) proposed competing legislation without a mandate for involuntary care. Neither bill left committee, and Murphy's legislation was reintroduced to Congress in 2015. In response to criticism of the earlier version, he had altered the bill so that states with outpatient commitment would receive more funds, rather than having the states without outpatient commitment lose funding, as the original legislation required.

While we believe that mass tragedies won't be prevented by mandating treatment for mental illness, we recognize that there are personal tragedies suffered by people with mental illness and their families every day in every community. Even if people with mental illness don't end up sleeping on the streets, or in jail or prison, or killing innocent people, mental illness leads to a loss of productivity and often diminishes the wonderful experience of being human. Legislation that provides funding for services to help people conquer such problems on their own terms—whether that is about getting through a difficult time or coping with a long-term and disabling psychotic disorder—makes all the sense in the world. Instead of mass murder, we'd prefer to focus on the second line of Murphy's quote in the *Guardian*: "And just as importantly, we can save countless lives of those with mental illness from suicide, victimization, homelessness and despair."

Psychiatric care both saves and enriches lives, and it seems a bit crazy that so much effort goes into forcing care when we don't allocate the resources to provide treatment to the many people who desperately want and need it.

Seven
FUTURE DIRECTIONS

It's a painful truth that medications and psychiatric hospitals, the faults of which could fill volumes, have both saved me, and made a good life for myself possible. For that, I am grateful.

—Mark Vonnegut, MD, on KevinMd.com,
June 19, 2015

S ome of the stories in this book are egregious examples of care gone wrong: a woman hospitalized involuntarily without a hearing for many weeks, a woman court-ordered to treatment when she was willing to get care voluntarily, and an accused murderer who spent years in a forensic hospital because he could not be either convinced or made to take the medications that might render him competent to stand trial. We believe these show a system gone awry. Imposing unwanted treatment without respect for civil rights or personal dignity, or withholding treatment in a way that leaves a person to suffer without relief, are both affronts to psychiatric ethics. Furthermore, US society has done a disgraceful job of providing voluntary care to its citizens, many of whom want the treatments that are being offered.

Voluntary care requires time and patience, both of which are in short supply. Convincing a patient to take medications can be challenging, and some psychiatric patients have issues that impair their insight as to their need for treatment. Now the media are saturated with stories about the dangers of psychotropic medications, how they are overprescribed, and how psychiatrists in particular have been unduly influenced by the pharmaceutical companies. Is it any wonder that patients might hesitate to take a pill and might need some time to make the decision?

When a patient is diagnosed with a curable cancer, a physician takes the time to discuss treatment options. Alternative regimens may be offered if the risk of one type of treatment is unacceptable to the patient. Even if the patient initially rejects all treatment, efforts are made to involve the family and to educate the patient about life-saving procedures. In psychiatry there is a similar need for building rapport. Kind and respectful care leads to trust and satisfaction with any type of medical treatment, including psychiatric treatment. Although a large number of people agree that involuntary treatment should be a last resort, health-care policies and institutions don't always agree on what "last resort" means and how much effort should go into the first resort of engaging people in voluntary treatment. Sometimes, involuntary treatment ends up being used as the *only* resort.

If you begin with the idea that psychiatric treatment is in the best interests of the patient—whether they recognize it or not during an episode of mental illness—then you do what is necessary to get that person help. You make treatment decisions with the idea that the end result of helping a very sick patient get better may be worth some indignities, and you hope that patients will later understand and appreciate that you've done what was needed to help them heal. Involuntary treatment then becomes a means to a desired end.

If you begin with the idea that involuntary psychiatric treatment might leave the patient feeling distressed and traumatized for years, then you start with a different mind-set and a different propensity to take action—especially action that might be viewed by an ill person as either a restriction of their rights or a physical assault. We'd like to refocus mental health professionals to consider this possibility: involuntary psychiatric care may be damaging. It may never be appreciated, and the fear of forced care may prevent people from seeking help.

If you begin with the idea that forced psychiatric care and its components—restriction of freedom, restraint, seclusion, forced medications—may traumatize patients, you still do it if someone's life is in danger. And you may still do it, though perhaps more gently, if their illness leaves them with intolerable suffering, even if there is not the imminent prospect of death or injury. However, if you start with the idea that involuntary care may be traumatizing, you do it much less often and much more thoughtfully.

Involuntary care is oversold because of the agendas of both psychiatrists and society: for cover-your-ass malpractice protection and as a means of "doing something" to prevent mass murders, agendas it simply can't fulfill.

Psychiatry has proven that it can make changes in its practices. We no longer use restraints with the misunderstanding that they are healing. We have dramatically decreased the use of both restraint and seclusion, and we have ended the use of long-term institutionalization as a routine method of warehousing patients.

In this conclusion, we recognize and support efforts to minimize indignity and suffering with the hope that the mental health battleground might be transformed into a conference table around which all voices are heard.

What follows are some suggestions we hope will promote psychiatric care that is more accessible and that is shaped by the values and preferences of our patients. Unfortunately, we don't foresee a way in the immediate future to eliminate all involuntary care.

An advance directive is a legal document that a patient can use to designate someone to make health-care decisions if he or she loses the ability to make decisions. A directive can specify which medications a patient prefers, which facility the patient wishes to be admitted to, and even who should care for the patient's children during a hospitalization. Eleanor was fortunate that she only had one psychotic episode, but the experience was so terrifying that she was fearful of another admission. Since she has a loving and supportive husband, as well as an outpatient psychiatrist she trusts, some of her fears might be eased by creating a directive that her outpatient doctor and inpatient team would follow in the event of a psychotic relapse. Jim, the patient who had involuntary ECT, created a document similar to an advance directive to guide his care. He designated his sister to have power of attorney and to give consent to treatment when he was unable to do so. People interested in this option can visit the website of the National Resource Center on Psychiatric Advance Directives for more information about each state's advance directive laws. The Bazelon Center website also offers templates for an advance directive document.

Presently, psychiatric advance directives cannot be used to refuse admission or to prevent civil commitment. For involuntarily admitted patients, we believe an admission standard based on dangerousness as a result of psychiatric illness is reasonable. In assessing dangerousness, a broad definition is necessary. Society must be protected from a mentally ill person who has committed a recent, overt act of violence, and a psychotic person should not be left to freeze or starve on the street. There are too many hypothetical situations for the law to anticipate them all, but we believe that the due process protections of a civil commitment hearing should allow for vigorous patient representation and an opportunity for patients to tell their side of the story. Many of the patients we interviewed for this book said that their hearings were perfunctory, with little regard for their input or without any input from them at all. This must change. Additionally, commitment hearings should respect individual privacy and should be held in a hospital rather than in an open courthouse.

The patients described certain hospital policies that were humiliating and arbitrary. We heard patients talk about the distress of strip searches, for example. While we don't know the prevalence of strip searches in psychiatric units in US hospitals today, it is certainly not a standard practice for all hospitals, and as a blanket policy for all patients who are admitted, it should be stopped. An inpatient unit is not a correctional facility, and patients are inherently due more rights and respect than are people accused of criminal acts.

Some patients also experienced deprivations that would be considered outrageous if inflicted upon a medically ill person, such as being left in the emergency room for long periods without access to family, food, water, and restroom facilities. A patient who experiences this type of treatment should have a mechanism to report it without fear of repercussion during a future admission, and a facility should be held accountable by accrediting agencies for such poor care.

We endorse efforts to train inpatient staff and emergency room personnel in the use of verbal de-escalation techniques. Where possible, patients should be allowed to develop their own de-escalation plan and to educate the staff regarding their particular violence triggers and calming techniques. We do not support a one-size-fits-all approach to the management of inpatient violence, nor do we recommend the use of a seclusion room or physical restraints as a first intervention for a patient who appears to be upset. The psychiatrists we interviewed were able to reduce inpatient violence using this alternative approach, although this gentler policy is more costly in terms of human resources and staff time. Since hospital accreditation agencies mandate efforts to reduce seclusion and restraint, insurance companies and government agencies should provide financial support for the additional staff required to accomplish this.

Crisis intervention training should be a mandatory and routine component of training for all correctional officers and all state and city police forces, rather than limiting this training to a handpicked and finite team of specialized officers in a limited number of localities. Training to recognize signs of mental illness and training in nonlethal interventions can circumvent the use of physical force. While the police have the right to be safe while interacting with unpredictable and agitated patients, handcuffing patients who are brought to the hospital by police should not be standard practice. Ideally, every jurisdiction should have a mobile crisis team, with a trained mental health professional to provide on-site consultation in emergency situations. Where arrest cannot be prevented, we support the creation of mental health courts and pretrial diversion services to shorten the length of incarceration pending trial and to tie a defendant more closely to needed community services.

The closure of state institutions and the loss of psychiatric hospital beds have created an unacceptable barrier to voluntary care. Nevertheless, we don't seek to reverse deinstitutionalization. Long-term hospitalization is no substitute for thoughtful community care. Intermediate levels of care should be more readily available to those who don't require admission but who need more intensive support than can be provided in the usual outpatient clinic setting. We agree with Ira Burnim of the Bazelon Center and with Ron Honberg of NAMI that there should be expanded use of mobile treatment teams, assertive community outreach, crisis centers, peer support services, patient-directed care initiatives, and a variety of housing options. We would extend this community service initiative to include suicide prevention hotlines, which need to be available to everyone and which should be widely publicized. Even where these services exist now, patients and their clinicians are often unaware of them.

Every system transformation requires some education and training for those providing services and for those in need of them. We believe there should be more intensive efforts to detect serious mental illness in its early stages. Too often the family and friends of a mentally ill teenager write off emerging symptoms of psychosis as normal adolescent turmoil or as the transient stress of young adulthood. Public education about the early signs of psychosis may enable patients to access services before a crisis occurs. Since most psychiatric care is provided by primary care physicians and other nonpsychiatrists, these professionals also need training to recognize and treat emerging mental disorders, and to recognize conditions that should be referred to a psychiatrist. In many cases, involuntary treatment could be avoided if care were available earlier in an episode of illness.

Sadly, the funding for training in psychiatry and its subspecialties has not kept up with the demand for these services. Medicare funding limits the number of doctors that can be trained at any particular teaching hospital, and that limit has not been raised since 1997. According to the US Department of Health and Human Services, the need for psychiatrists is expected to increase by 16 percent by 2020, but this demand is not going to be met by current training programs. There should be increased government support for psychiatric training, as well as more opportunities for student loan forgiveness for psychiatrists who work in underserved areas.

In chapter 4, we interviewed Daniel Fisher, who had been hospitalized several times between 1969 and 1974. He specifically mentioned the distress of being given "mind-numbing medication." We have many more medications available today, which work equally well with fewer side effects, but even these newer medications carry risks. The discovery of penicillin was a miraculous cure for many infectious diseases, but psychiatry has had no analogous miracle. We need to keep searching for better treatments, either medications or other interventions, that will cure disease rather than merely control symptoms.

Presently, the funding for innovation in psychiatry is primarily reliant on for-profit industries rather than independent research grants. Traditionally, medical journals have been biased in favor of research that shows that medications work and have not published studies that show medications to be ineffective. This publication bias may lead people to believe that a new medication is more efficacious than it really is in practice. Patients also suffer when the cost of an effective medication is exorbitant. Financial incentives encourage drug manufacturers to abandon effective older treatments when a newer medication is more lucrative. The best way to change this situation and ensure independent research is to enrich government-sponsored basic science and clinical research. The National Institute of Mental Health is the largest government sponsor of psychiatric research in the United States, yet its budget has not kept up with inflation in the twenty-first century. The NIMH is currently able to fund only 20 percent of its annual grant applications. There needs to be more government-sponsored—independent—financial support for the treatment of psychiatric illnesses.

Finally, we recognize that, in spite of our best efforts, there will be a small number of people who are both violent and mentally ill. For these patients, we support psychiatrists who work in public institutions, such as jails, prisons, and forensic hospitals. It is not possible to separate human beings cleanly into the "mad" versus the "bad." Even with programs in place to divert misdemeanor or nonviolent offenders, there will always be a need for correctional mental health services. Improvement of correctional mental health services should not have to depend on class action litigation or the media pressure that follows a high-profile jail suicide. Close community supervision is also necessary, and we support efforts to integrate jail or prison release plans, with state correctional institutions and public mental health systems working together.

While we don't support laws that restrict civil rights based solely on the existence of a mental health diagnosis or a history of mental health treatment, we do support restricting the gun rights of anyone with a history of violent behavior, including suicide attempts, and active alcohol and drug abuse issues. In addition, we support the use of emergency gun restraining orders with anyone who is threatening violence. We support laws that require the safe storage of firearms; limitations on assault weapons, stockpiles of ammunition, and arsenals of firearms; and requirements for licensing, registration, and training. When the technology becomes available for "smart guns," which recognize their lawful owners, we think this may be helpful in preventing accidental deaths and the transfer of weapons to those who are disqualified from owning them.

There is a common theme to many of these recommendations: they require money. Fortunately, the Affordable Care Act (ACA) is being implemented across the United States. The ACA is a controversial law with mixed blessings; it creates administrative mandates that divert physician time away from patient care, but it also increases access to care by providing federal funding for previously uninsured people, including people with mental illness. It encourages the creation of so-called medical homes, which provide an integrated system of medical care, including mental health and substance abuse services, in addition to traditional medical services.

Some early results from the use of this model of care have been promising. In 2007, the Harris County jail created a project to link Houston's homeless mentally ill prisoners with community services upon release, using the medical home model. The project linked the detainee with community mental health, medical, and substance abuse services in addition to addressing housing and transportation needs. After three years the project demonstrated that more than half the released prisoners stayed in treatment and that criminal charges dropped by more than 50 percent in the year following engagement in the program. It may well be that the most effective way to reduce both crime and involuntary care will come through the innovations created with the ACA. With enough government foresight, the savings realized from decreased incarceration could be used for psychiatric research and education.

Involuntary treatment needs to be limited to situations where the *only* agenda is the best interest of the patient after other options to engage the patient have been exhausted. In any discussion of eliminating involuntary care, we need to remember that there are patients like Lily: she was miserable with her delusions and was grateful for the involuntary treatment she received. It's a daunting, if not impossible, task to figure out how to preserve one person's right to refuse unwanted treatment while preserving another person's right to get well when they aren't able to negotiate their own way.

The above conclusions come from both of us, as co-authors, after years of research, consideration, and heated discussion. For just a moment, Dr. Miller wants to break from our joint summary and share an anecdote about how this research has influenced her personal practice of clinical psychiatry.

In the course of writing this book, I came to believe that involuntary treatment could be damaging and should be avoided whenever possible. I have spent more than 20 years working in four different community mental health centers in the greater Baltimore area. In addition, I've had a private practice in a state without laws for mandated outpatient care; in this setting, involuntary treatment is a rare event. Still, there have been times when I became deeply concerned about the safety of several of my patients. In these cases, the patients refused voluntary hospitalization.

Believing that forced care could be traumatizing, I tried other methods to avoid involuntary treatment. When possible, I involved family members, and I had daily contact and frequent appointments with the patients I was concerned about. I wondered—and I still wonder—if my work on this book clouded my judgment and endangered my patients. In the end, no one was injured, and no one said they wished I'd had the police haul them off to a hospital, but the truth is that if anyone had died, my stance would have been unforgivable. I lost sleep over these cases, and I still feel a little queasy when I think about how high the stakes were.

I have come to appreciate how much easier these decisions are in hindsight, after a crisis has passed, or as an abstract theory when human lives are not involved. Without a crystal ball to guide us, and with the knowledge that bad outcomes certainly do occur, it's simply not possible to write a script with exact guidelines for what to do when the question comes up about usurping a patient's autonomy. The correct answer only is clear in retrospect. It's not always obvious, even to the most experienced of psychiatrists, what is the right thing to do while trying to predict another human being's behavior.

Our recommendations are made based on our combined professional experience as well as the problems we've come to appreciate while writing this book. We are still left with gaps in our knowledge. We don't know how often people who want treatment are unable to obtain voluntary care nor do we know the number of tragedies that have resulted from this lack of care. When it comes to involuntary treatments, we don't know how often people feel traumatized, or helped, or what can be done to minimize the distress of those who feel violated. These open questions we leave to our readers. We hope that this book inspires action on the part of the US government and our profession, action that will ultimately offer comfort to patients and their loved ones.

Acknowledgments

Dinah Miller

This book has been about more than writing a book; it's been a major project that has captivated my thinking for a number of years. Many people were drawn in voluntarily, others with a bit of coercion (or even hijacked) into my world to help with this, and I have a long list of people to thank who so generously shared their time, their knowledge, and their experiences with me.

Ray DePaulo has been a constant source of support and encouragement, and he allowed me to shadow him on an inpatient unit at Johns Hopkins Hospital at a time when no one else wanted a psychiatrist-journalist on their psychiatry units. Ray literally saved this project just as I thought it would need to be abandoned. After I could say that the chairman of the Department of Psychiatry at Johns Hopkins was a willing participant, the project gained a degree of credibility, and future doors opened more easily. I can't thank him enough.

Jeff Swanson is a brilliant researcher who possesses an enormous fund of knowledge about things I find fascinating: guns, mental health, violence, and outpatient civil commitment. He was kind, patient, and generous with his knowledge, and he sent long answers to my many emails, often including papers that were still in press and information that no one else had. On the rare occasions when he didn't have an answer, he knew who did. Jeff was instrumental in supporting the creation of this book.

Fuller Torrey and I don't exactly agree on all aspects of involuntary treatment, but still, he was kind, patient, responsive, and willing to help. His input added a tremendous amount to this book, and I hope I captured his passionate, colorful, and provocative persona. No one else has ever asked me if I wanted a mentally ill spree shooter to be my next-door neighbor.

Paul Appelbaum was also kind and responsive and served as a resource for pretty much anything that someone else didn't know. The scope of his knowledge is astounding.

The patients who contributed to this book brought it to life. I can't thank "Eleanor" and "Lily" enough for all the hours of their time and for opening their hearts to me, for allowing me to speak with their doctors and families, and for giving me access to their medical records. Without these two women, this book simply could not have happened. I asked for just a little less from "Jim," his sister "Ella," "Marsha," "Amy," "Elizabeth," and "Sherry"—who all shared their stories with the hope of helping others. In addition to the accounts I used in the book, I spoke with many more people all over the United States about their experiences with involuntary care. Journalist Pete Earley recruited people for me on his popular advocacy website, and psychiatrist-author Mark Komrad asked his patients who had been involuntarily treated if they would tell me their stories. I want to express my heartfelt gratitude to all of these people, who were willing to revisit some of the most painful memories of their lives to help with this book. None of this was easy.

There are accounts included here that we simply lifted from the media, and we did not contact the patients, their families, or their victims: those that entailed heinous crimes, mass murders, and the deaths of both strangers and loved ones. The people who have suffered because of an untreated or undertreated mental illness all deserve acknowledgment. We're hoping for a kinder, gentler, more available, and more effective psychiatry in the future. Many people are mentioned in the chapters, and many people guided me. In no particular order, I want to thank Ron Honberg, Ira Burnim, Celia Brown, Janet Foner, "Bob" (the Christian Scientologist), Dan Fisher, Paul Summergrad, Steven Sharfstein, Bob Roca, Erik Roskes, Brian Hepburn, "Leonard Skivorski," Jeff Janofsky, Phil Cronin, Bryce Hewitt, Marvin Bernstein, Bob Bernstein, Chris Devaney, Henry Dlugacz, Ryan Bell, Adam Nelson, Jerry Lazar, Jerry Gallucci, Stephen Dettwyler, Kevin Klauer, Bruce Hershfield, Jack Lesser, Charlotte Cooksey, Kathleen Sweeney (who inspired both Judge Lesser and Judge Cooksey to speak to me), the amazing staff of the Baltimore City Mental Health Court, Scott Davis, Betsy Davis, Rob Bossarte, Marsden McGuire (who led me to Rob Bossarte), Adam Rosenblatt (who *invited* me to visit his unit and spent his afternoon off hosting a tour of the facilities), Ananda Pandurangi, Glenn Miller, John Marcos, a psychiatrist in Texas who wished to remain unnamed, Steve Leifman, Harvey Rosenthal, Kim Butler, the staff of Meyer 3 (who tolerated having me there, sometimes not quite as quietly as I'd promised I'd be, for a week in the winter of 2014), Barbara Schweitzer (who helped negotiate the HIPAA compliance of my visit), the staff at the Medical College of Virginia ECT suite, Dom Sisti (whom I befriended at the Scattergood ethics conference), Candice Player, John Monahan, Angela Guarda, Irving Reti, Phil Ross, Steve Daviss, Joshua Sonkiss, Margaret Bolton, and Elyn Saks. Even with this lengthy list, I'm thinking there must still be many people I've forgotten. I'm grateful to you all.

My family—David, Rachel, and Jerry—and all of my close friends listened to countless hours of my excited chatter about involuntary psychiatric treatment. Thank you to Sally and Henry, Kathleen, Carol, Maria, Jesse and Debby, Steve and Barb, Emile, Hinda, Susan and Robert, Cousin Barb and Fred, Rich and Vicki, Linda, and everyone else who listened. Even my mother-in-law, Elise Donabedian, was held hostage on the topic. I "offered" a chapter to read, and she did so voluntarily, I think. Pete Earley and David Brown were both incredible when I needed the wisdom of real journalists. David was kind enough to read and critique a large chunk of the manuscript, an enormous favor I hope to somehow be able to repay.

Ramin Mojtabai was patient, listening to my random ideas over time. He insisted—repeatedly—that I had to read Lonny Shavelson's book *Hooked*. I finally did, and it was through *Hooked* that I found our literary agent, Felicia Eth, to represent *Committed*. It was a long process to give this project its full definition, and Felicia was both tremendously patient and invested. She was even gracious about the daily emails I sent with links to articles about involuntary psychiatric care from newspapers around the country.

Jackie Wehmueller, the executive editor at Johns Hopkins University Press, is both an amazing editor and a wonderful friend. Sometimes I can beat her at Words with Friends, and for that and many other things, I am so grateful. She has come to be an important person in my life over the course of two books now.

Finally, I can't thank my co-author, Anne Hanson, enough for putting up with my projects over the decades and for getting excited about the battle over forced psychiatric care along with me. While I was out talking with fascinating people, she was behind the scenes doing an amazing job of reviewing and summarizing the literature; she also told me about Oxford commas, among many other things. In addition to being a walking encyclopedia of forensic psychiatry, Annie provided support, encouragement, and companionship during this entire endeavor. We've developed a rhythm for writing together, a way of coming to consensus (sometimes even painlessly), and her friendship has made writing—which can be a lonely adventure—so much more enjoyable. No one has ever had a better partner in psychiatric writing.

Annette Hanson

I would like to thank all those who fostered my interest in forensic psychiatry and helped with this book, in no particular order of appearance, preference, or degree of influence, including Doctors Jeff Janofsky, Jonas Rappeport, Christiane Tellefsen, and Paul Appelbaum. Thank you all for your brilliance and good humor. Dr. Rebecca Birnbaum and the Academy of Psychiatry and the Law were kind enough to grant permission to quote extensively from "My Father's Advocacy for a Right to Treatment." I thank Nicholas P. Conti, LCSW-C, for teaching me how the forensic and judicial systems really work—and how to manage them when they don't. Special thanks to Dr. Khalid El-Sayed for sharing my workload so that this manuscript could be finished by our self-imposed deadline, and to Dr. Dan Marshall for boosting my morale through his mastery of Internet cat memes. Perhaps someday I will be able to return the favor. I join Dinah in thanking our editor, Jackie Wehmueller, for being a gentle mediator. I don't know how she's put up with both of us for all these years.

My colleagues, friends, and students at the Clifton T. Perkins Hospital Center kindly listened to me vent, which carried me through the rough patches of the writing process. The list is too long to mention them all, but I am constantly impressed by their dedication. I hope that this book will help the general public understand the challenges that clinical staff face every day while caring for very ill, potentially dangerous patients. Similarly, I'd like to recognize my colleagues in the Psychology Department at the Maryland Reception Diagnostic and Classification Center for continuing to provide badly needed mental health services to prisoners during a time of citywide disruption and violence. You are all heroes.

Writing this book was no easy task. Dinah and I differ in personality, in cognitive style, and in our writing methods. In order to produce a unified voice, I agreed to remain the silent partner and did not inject myself into the body of the work; except for one chapter, the voice expressed in this book is almost entirely hers. Where there are shortcomings in the literature review, the research summaries, or the historical background material, the fault is mine.

Dinah and I have had very different professional experiences, and we have worked with very different patient populations. My patients and evaluees are all institutionalized, are involved in the criminal justice system, and for the most part have few resources or social supports. Some of them have been violent. Dinah's patients are not all so disadvantaged, and it came as no surprise that we sometimes had differences in our approach to involuntary treatment. How we managed these differences is illustrative; even though we bickered at times, we still were able to hammer out our conflicts, and we remained friends. This process was emblematic of the theme of this book; we began with a mental health system battleground but ended with unity and agreed-upon solutions. Given that the health and well-being of our patients is at stake, I hope the factions discussed in this book will also be willing to face their conflicts for the sake of unity. Even if it's sometimes necessary that you shout to be taken seriously, we silent partners in psychiatry do listen. We wrote this book because we heard you.

References

Before We Get Started

Now Is the Time: The President's Plan to Protect Our Children and Our Communities by Reducing Gun Violence. January 16, 2013. www.whitehouse.gov/sites/default/files/docs/wh_now_is_the_time_full.pdf.

New York SAFE Act. http://www.omh.ny.gov/omhweb/safe_act/.

US Government. www.Data.gov.

Torrey, E. F., D. A. Fuller, J. Geller, C. Jacobs, and K. Rogosta. "No Room at the Inn: Trends and Consequences of Closing Public Psychiatric Hospitals 2005–2010." Report by Treatment Advocacy Center, 2012. http://tacreports.org/bed-study.

2. Lily and the Case for Civil Commitment

Ohio Revised Code Annotated 5122.01(B), 5122.10. http://codes.ohio.gov/orc/5122.01. Accessed January 24, 2016.

Social Security. "What Can Cause Disability Benefits to Stop." http://www.ssa.gov/dibplan/dwork2.htm.

Protection and Advocacy for Mentally Ill Individuals Act—Systems Required. 42 US Code § 15043.

3. In Favor of Involuntary Treatments

St. Elizabeths Hospital. https://en.wikipedia.org/wiki/St._Elizabeths_Hospital.

Torrey, E. F., D. A. Fuller, J. Geller, C. Jacobs, and K. Rogosta. "No Room at the Inn: Trends and Consequences of Closing Public Psychiatric Hospitals 2005–2010." Report by Treatment Advocacy Center, 2012. http://tacreports.org/bed-study.

National Alliance on Mental Illness. www.NAMI.org.

Whitaker, Robert. *Anatomy of an Epidemic: Magic Bullets, Psychiatric Drugs, and the Astonishing Rise of Mental Illness in America.* Broadway Books, 2011.

Earley, Pete. "Whitaker: Has NAMI Opened a Pandora's Box?" July 5, 2013. http://www.peteearley.com/2013/07/05/whitaker-has-nami-opened-a-pandoras-box/.

4. Against Involuntary Treatments

Citizens Commission on Human Rights International. http://www.cchrint.org.

Thomas S. Szasz Cybercenter for Liberty and Responsibility. http://www.szasz.com /intro.html.

Interview of Thomas Szasz. http://www.szasz.com/lastthreemin.mov.

MindFreedom International. http://www.mindfreedom.org/.

Oaks, David. "MindFreedom Intro, Part One." https://www.youtube.com/watch ?v=bZSB90dFSNg.

Fisher, Daniel. *My Story*. http://akmhcweb.org/recovery/My_Story.htm.

Fisher, Daniel. Speech in front of the Boston State House, June 2, 2012. http:// www.madinamerica.com/2012/06/are-we-not-human-beings-with-the-rights -to-be-treated-as-human/.

National Empowerment Center. http://www.power2u.org/who.htm.

Long, Liza. "5 Reasons I Wish We Would Stop Talking about 'Recovery' for Serious Mental Illness and the Word I Wish We Would Use Instead." *Huffington Post*, January 30, 2015.

Bazelon Center. http://www.bazelon.org/Who-We-Are/History.aspx.

5. Eleanor, Lily, and the Process of Civil Commitment

Bruckner, Tim A., Jangho Yoon, Timothy T. Brown, and Neal Adams. "Involuntary Civil Commitments after the Implementation of California's Mental Health Services Act." *Psychiatric Services* (October 1, 2010): 1006-11.

Lanterman-Petris-Short Act. California Welfare and Institutions Code. http:// ca.regstoday.com/law/wic/ca.regstoday.com/laws/wic/calaw-wic_DIVISION 5_PART1_CHAPTER2.aspx#1.

Superior Court of California, County of Los Angeles. "What Is a LPS Hold?" http://www.lacourt.org/division/mentalhealth/MH0018.aspx.

Ohio Revised Code Annotated 5122.01(B), 5122.10. http://codes.ohio.gov/orc /5122.01 Accessed January 24, 2016.

Sonkiss, Joshua. Unpublished action paper proposed to the American Psychiatric Association, 2015.

"Shame of the City: Homeless in San Francisco." *SFGate*. http://www.sfgate.com /homeless. Accessed February 2, 2016.

Appelbaum, Paul S., and Thomas G. Gutheil. "'Rotting with Their Rights On': Constitutional Theory and Clinical Reality in Drug Refusal by Psychiatric Patients." *Bulletin of the American Academy of Psychiatry and the Law* 7, no. 3 (1979): 306–15.

6. Christina Schumacher and the History of Civil Commitment Laws

Schumacher, Christina. Video of public testimony to Vermont legislators, January 2014. *Burlington Free Press*. http://www.burlingtonfreepress.com/story/news /2014/01/30/schumacher-addresses-state-senate-on-involuntary-hospitalizat ion/5066485.

Donoghue, Mike. "Police: Essex Student Slain More than 24 Hours before Body Found." *Burlington Free Press*, December 19, 2013.

Donoghue, Mike. "Judge: Release Christina Schumacher Immediately." *Burlington Free Press*, January 24, 2014.

Donoghue, Mike."Schumacher Rewrote Will before Murder-Suicide." *Burlington Free Press*, February 14, 2014.

Goodnough, Abby. "Storm Has Vermont Scrambling to Find Beds for Mentally Ill." *New York Times*, November 4, 2011.

"Project Aids Those in Involuntary Mental Health System." Vermont Public Radio, January 10, 2013.

Unger, Ron. "I Got Better: MindFreedom's New Campaign to Fight Misinformation with Personal Stories." June 14, 2012. http://recoveryfromschizophrenia.org/2012 /06/i-got-better-mindfreedoms-new-campaign-to-fight-misinformation-with -personal-stories.

"History of Pennsylvania Hospital." http://www.uphs.upenn.edu/paharc/timeline /1751/.

Packard, E. P. W. *The Prisoners' Hidden Life; or, Insane Asylums Unveiled*. Chicago: A. B. Case, 1868.

Lake v. Cameron. 364 F.2d 657 (1966).

Lessard v. Schmidt. 349 F.Supp. 1078 (1972).

O'Connor v. Donaldson. 422 US 563 (1975).

Birnbaum, Rebecca. "My Father's Advocacy for a Right to Treatment." *Journal of the American Academy of Psychiatry and the Law* 38, no. 1 (2010): 115–23.

Protection and Advocacy for Mentally Ill Individuals Act—Systems Required. 42 US Code § 15043.

Fasulo v. Arafeh. 378 A.2d 553 (1977).

7. Scott Davis on Law Enforcement and Crisis Intervention Teams

US Census Bureau. "State and County QuickFacts." http://quickfacts.census.gov /qfd/states/24/24031.html.

Crisis Services, Montgomery County, Maryland. http://www.montgomerycounty md.gov/HHS-Program/Program.aspx?id=BHCS/BHCSAdultmentalhealth -p321.html.

Warner, Dudley. Presentation on crisis services. Maryland DHMH Outpatient Services Programs workgroup meeting, June 24, 2014.

Health—General. Maryland Code Annotated § 10-613. https://www.lexisnexis.com /hottopics/mdcode. Accessed January 24, 2016.

Boscarato, Kara, Stuart Lee, Jon Kroschel, Yitzchak Hollander, Alice Brennan, and Narelle Warren. "Consumer Experience of Formal Crisis-Response Services and Preferred Methods of Crisis Intervention." *International Journal of Mental Health Nursing* (February 27, 2014). doi:10.1111/inm.12059.

Memphis Model. Memphis Police Department. http://www.memphispolice.org /crisis%20intervention.htm.

Compton, Michael T., et al. "A Comprehensive Review of Extant Research on Crisis Intervention Team (CIT) Programs." *Journal of the American Academy of Psychiatry and the Law* 36, no. 1 (2008): 47–55.

Compton, Michael T., et al. "System- and Policy-Level Challenges to Full Implementation of the Crisis Intervention Team (CIT) Model." *Journal of Police Crisis Negotiations: An International Journal* 10, nos. 1–2 (2010): 72–85. doi:10.1080/15332581003757347.

Compton, Michael T., et al. "Do Empathy and Psychological Mindedness Affect Police Officers' Decision to Enter Crisis Intervention Team Training?" *Psychiatric Services (Washington, D.C.)* 62, no. 6 (June 2011): 632–38. doi:10.1176/appi.ps.62 .6.632.

Compton, Michael T., et al. "The Police-Based Crisis Intervention Team (CIT) Model: I. Effects on Officers' Knowledge, Attitudes, and Skills." *Psychiatric Services (Washington, D.C.)* 65, no. 4 (April 2014): 517–22. doi:10.1176/appi.ps.201300107.

Compton, Michael T., et al. "The Police-Based Crisis Intervention Team (CIT) Model: II. Effects on Level of Force and Resolution, Referral, and Arrest." *Psychiatric Services (Washington, D.C.)* 65, no. 4 (April 2014): 523–29. doi:10.1176 /appi.ps.201300108.

Federal Bureau of Investigation. *Law Enforcement Officers Killed and Assaulted.* 2012. http://www.fbi.gov/about-us/cjis/ucr/leoka/2012/officers-feloniously-killed /felonious_topic_page_-2012.

Amnesty International. "Concerns about Taser Use: Statement to the US Justice Department Inquiry into Deaths in Custody." October 2007. http://cdm16064 .contentdm.oclc.org/cdm/ref/collection/p266901coll4/id/2853.

Leifman, Steve. Speech for the Productive Lives Award, Brain and Behavior Research Foundation. 2012. https://www.youtube.com/watch?v=UM5vQFn3ij4.

Warner, Dudley. Presentation on crisis services. Maryland DHMH Outpatient Services Programs workgroup meeting, June 24, 2014.

Bureau of Justice Statistics. "Police Behavior during Traffic and Street Stops." 2011. NCJ 242937. http://www.bjs.gov/content/pub/pdf/pbtss11.pdf.

8. Leonard Skivorski and the Emergency Department

Kirk, Stuart A., Tomi Gomory, and David Cohen. *Mad Science: Psychiatric Coercion, Diagnosis, and Drugs.* Transaction Publishers, 2013.

Malowney, Monica, Sarah Keltz, Daniel Fischer, and J. Wesley Boyd. "Availability of Outpatient Care from Psychiatrists: A Simulated-Patient Study in Three U.S. Cities." *Psychiatric Services* 66, no. 1 (January 2015): 94–96.

Sun, Lena H. "Why It's So Hard to Find a Mental Health Professional." *Washington Post*, October 22, 2015.

Earley, Pete. *Crazy: A Father's Search through America's Mental Health Madness.* Penguin, 2007.

Hancock, Daniel, Johnson, and Nagel, PC. "Virginia's Changing Mental Health Laws." Client advisory, April 30, 2008.

Glatter, Robert. "'Boarding' of Psychiatric Patients in Emergency Rooms Unconstitutional in Washington State." *Forbes*, August 16, 2014.

Taylor-Desir, Monica. "Civil Commitment: Assessment of Statutes of Area 7 States and Native Sovereign Nations." Paper presented at the American Psychiatric Association annual meeting, May 19, 2015.

9. Eleanor's Hospital Experience

Holland, Julie. *Weekends at Bellevue: Nine Years on the Night Shift at the Psych ER*. Bantam, 2009.

Insel, Thomas. "Antipsychotics: Taking the Long View." NIMH director's blog. August 28, 2013. http://www.nimh.nih.gov/about/director/2013/antipsychotics -taking-the-long-view.shtml.

Andreasen, Nancy C., Dawei Liu, Steven Ziebell, Anvi Vora, and Beng-Choon Ho. "Relapse Duration, Treatment Intensity, and Brain Tissue Loss in Schizophrenia: A Prospective Longitudinal MRI Study." *American Journal of Psychiatry* 170 (2013): 609–15. doi:10.1176/appi.ajp.2013.12050674.

Breggin, Peter. *Medication Madness: The Role of Psychiatric Drugs in Cases of Violence, Suicide and Murder*. St. Martin's Press, 2008.

10. Ray DePaulo and Inpatient Psychiatry at a University Hospital

US News and World Report. "Health." http://health.usnews.com/best-hospitals /rankings/psychiatry. Accessed January 31, 2016.

Komrad, Mark S. *You Need Help! A Step-by-Step Plan to Convince a Loved One to Get Counseling*. Hazelden, 2012.

11. Steven Sharfstein, Bruce Hershfield, and Free-Standing Psychiatric Hospitals

Sharfstein, Steven, MD. Testimony before the Maryland Senate Finance Committee, February 26, 2014.

Ebeling, Bill. "A Brief History of Springfield Hospital Center." Maryland Department of Health and Mental Hygiene. http://www.dhmh.maryland.gov /springfield/SitePages/history.aspx.

US News and World Report. "Health." http://health.usnews.com/best-hospitals /rankings/psychiatry. Accessed January 31, 2016.

12. Annette Hanson and the Use of Seclusion and Restraint

Weiss, E. M., et al. "Deadly Restraint: A Hartford Courant Investigative Report." *Hartford Courant*, October 11–15, 1998. http://www.charlydmiller.com/LIB05 /1998hartfordcourant11.html.

"Hospital Conditions of Participation: Patients' Rights; Final Rule." 71 *Federal Register* 236 (December 8, 2006): 71378–428.

Mental Health Systems Act of 1980. 42 US Code § 9501.

"Minnesota Security Hospital: Staff in Crisis Spreads Turmoil." *Minneapolis Star-Tribune*, January 1, 2014. http://www.startribune.com/lifestyle/health/237438721 .html.

Public Health and Welfare. Requirement Relating to the Rights of Residents of Certain Facilities: Regulations and Enforcement. 42 US Code § 290ii.

"Press Release: Data from Inpatient Psychiatric Facilities Increase Transparency for Consumers Evaluating Facilities." Centers for Medicare and Medicaid Services. April 17, 2014. http://www.cms.gov/Newsroom/MediaReleaseDatabase/Press -releases/2014-Press-releases-items/2014-04-17.html.

De Benedictis, Luigi, et al. "Staff Perceptions and Organizational Factors as Predictors of Seclusion and Restraint on Psychiatric Wards." *Psychiatric Services (Washington, D.C.)* 62, no. 5 (May 2011): 484-91. doi:10.1176/appi.ps.62.5.484.

Rezendes, Michael. "Bridgewater State Hospital Slow to Embrace Change." *Boston Globe*, June 1, 2014. https://www.bostonglobe.com/metro/2014/05/31/while -other-mental-health-facilities-cut-back-bridgewater-state-hospital-increased-use -harsh-tactics-patients/cdyiEwDddNdyv9qM9e4tSI/story.html.

Betemps, E. J., E. Somoza, and C. R. Buncher. "Hospital Characteristics, Diagnoses, and Staff Reasons Associated with Use of Seclusion and Restraint." *Hospital and Community Psychiatry* 44, no. 4 (April 1993): 367–71.

Frueh, B. Christopher, et al. "Patients' Reports of Traumatic or Harmful Experiences within the Psychiatric Setting." *Psychiatric Services* 56, no. 9 (September 2005): 1123–33.

Saks, Elyn R. *The Center Cannot Hold: My Journey through Madness*. Hachette Books, 2007.

Romney, L. "Atascadero Psychiatric Patient Arrested in Slaying of Fellow Patient." *Los Angeles Times*. May 29, 2014. http://www.latimes.com/local/lanow/la-me-ln -atascadero-patient-arrest-20140529-story.html.

McEnroe, P. "Patient at St. Peter Hospital Charged with Murder in Killing of Another Patient." *Minneapolis Star Tribune*. January 24, 2014. http://www.star tribune.com/local/241908761.html.

Protection and Advocacy for Individuals with Mental Illness Act of 1986. 42 US Code § 10801.

Smith, Gregory M., et al. "Pennsylvania State Hospital System's Seclusion and Restraint Reduction Program." *Psychiatric Services* 56, no. 9 (September 2005): 1115–22.

13. Anthony Kelly and Involuntary Medications

Riese v. St. Mary's Hospital and Medical Center. 259 Cal. Rptr. 669, 774 P.2d 698 (1989).

Department of Health and Mental Hygiene. Amicus brief no. 02227, *Department of Health & Mental Hygiene v. Anthony Kelly*. http://psychrights.org/states/Mary land/AGStatevKellyBrief.pdf. Accessed July 13, 2015.

Department of Health & Mental Hygiene v. Kelly. 397 Md. 399 (2007).

Rolon, Yamilka M., and Joshua C. W. Jones. "Right to Refuse Treatment." *Journal of the American Academy of Psychiatry and the Law* 36, no. 2 (2008): 252–55.

Morse, Dan. "Man Found Guilty of Killing Girl, Father." *Washington Post*, August 5, 2008.

Tucker, Neely. "A Case and a Survivor Come Out of an Abyss." *Washington Post*, January 21, 2010.

Sharfstein, Steven, MD. Testimony before the Maryland Senate Finance Committee, February 26, 2014.

Raines, Linda. Testimony before the Maryland Senate Finance Committee, February 26, 2014.

Anonymous patient. Testimony before the Maryland Senate Finance Committee, February 26, 2014.

14. Jim and Involuntary Electroconvulsive Therapy

One Flew over the Cuckoo's Nest. Milos Forman, dir., 1975.

Hermann, R. C., R. A. Dorwart, C. W. Hoover, and J. Brody. "Variation in ECT Use in the United States." *American Journal of Psychiatry* 152, no. 6 (June 1995): 869–75.

Harris, Victoria. "Electroconvulsive Therapy: Administrative Codes, Legislation, and Professional Recommendations." *Journal of the American Academy of Psychiatry and the Law* 34, no. 3 (2006): 406–11.

Brown, D. "FDA Panel Advises More Testing of 'Shock-Therapy' Devices." *Washington Post*, January 28, 2011. http://www.washingtonpost.com/wp-dyn /content/article/2011/01/28/AR2011012806328.html.

"Your Gateway to Stop the FDA Rubberstamp of ECT." MindFreedom International. http://www.mindfreedom.org/campaign/shield/fda-ect/fda-ect -gateway.

15. Marsha and Outpatient Civil Commitment

US Department of Justice, Office of Public Affairs. "Justice Department Obtains Comprehensive Agreement regarding the State of Delaware's Mental Health System." July 6, 2011. http://www.justice.gov/opa/pr/justice-department-obtains -comprehensive-agreement-regarding-state-delawares-mental-health.

16. Outpatient Commitment on the Books

Harticollis, Anemone. "Nearly 7 Years Later, Guilty Plea in New York Subway Killing." *New York Times*, October 11, 2006.

New York State Office of Mental Health. "Implementation of Kendra's Law." https://www.omh.ny.gov/omhweb/Kendra_web/interimreport/implementation .htm. Accessed January 24, 2016.

New York State Office of Mental Health. "Final Report on the Status of Assisted Outpatient Treatment Resources to Provide Court-Ordered Services." http://www .omh.ny.gov/omhweb/kendra_web/finalreport/resources.htm. Accessed January 24, 2016.

New York State Office of Mental Health. "AOT Statistics in NY." http://bi.omh .ny.gov/aot/statistics?p=petitions-filed. Accessed January 24, 2016.

Appelbaum, P. S. "Thinking Carefully about Outpatient Commitment." *Psychiatric Services (Washington, D.C.)* 52, no. 3 (March 2001): 347–50.

Report by the Task Force on Involuntary Outpatient Commitment, American Psychiatric Association. 1987. http://www.psychiatry.org/file%20library/learn /archives/tfr1987_involuntarycommitment.pdf.

Brooks, Robert A. "Psychiatrists' Opinions about Involuntary Civil Commitment: Results of a National Survey." *Journal of the American Academy of Psychiatry and the Law* 35, no. 2 (2007): 219–28.

Bazelon Center for Mental Health Law. "Involuntary Outpatient Commitment: Summary of State Statutes." http://www.bazelon.org/LinkClick.aspx?fileticket=CBmFgyA4i-w%3d&tabid=324. Accessed July 15, 2015.

Glatter, Robert. "'Boarding' of Psychiatric Patients in Emergency Rooms Unconstitutional in Washington State." *Forbes*, August 16, 2014.

"Mass Shootings at Virginia Tech: Report of the Review Panel." April 16, 2007. https://governor.virginia.gov/media/3772/fullreport.pdf.

Torrey, E. F., and M. Zdanowicz. "Outpatient Commitment: What, Why, and for Whom." *Psychiatric Services (Washington, D.C.)* 52, no. 3 (2001): 337–41.

Kisely, Steve R., Leslie Anne Campbell, and Neil J. Preston. "Compulsory Community and Involuntary Outpatient Treatment for People with Severe Mental Disorders." *Cochrane Database of Systematic Reviews*, no. 2 (2011): CD004408. doi:10.1002/14651858.CD004408.pub3.

Bellevue Pilot Study. http://csipmh.rfmh.org/projects/ti2.htm. Accessed January 24, 2016.

Steadman, H. J., K. Gounis, D. Dennis, K. Hopper, B. Roche, M. Swartz, and P. C. Robbins. "Assessing the New York City Involuntary Outpatient Commitment Pilot Program." *Psychiatric Services (Washington, D.C.)* 52, no. 3 (March 2001): 330–36.

Swartz, M. S., J. W. Swanson, V. A. Hiday, H. R. Wagner, B. J. Burns, and R. Borum. "A Randomized Controlled Trial of Outpatient Commitment in North Carolina." *Psychiatric Services (Washington, D.C.)* 52, no. 3 (March 2001): 325–29.

Swartz, M. S., J. W. Swanson, H. J. Steadman, and J. Monahan. "New York State Assisted Outpatient Treatment Program Evaluation." New York State Office of Mental Health. 2009. https://www.omh.ny.gov/omhweb/resources/publications /aot_program_evaluation/report.pdf.

Cornwell, John Kip, and Raymond Deeney. "Exposing the Myths Surrounding Preventive Outpatient Commitment for Individuals with Chronic Mental Illness." *Psychology, Public Policy, and Law: An Official Law Review of the University of Arizona College of Law and the University of Miami School of Law* 9, nos. 1–2 (June 2003): 209–32.

Allen, M., and V. F. Smith. "Opening Pandora's Box: The Practical and Legal Dangers of Involuntary Outpatient Commitment." *Psychiatric Services (Washington, D.C.)* 52, no. 3 (March 2001): 342–46.

Gerbasi, J. B., R. J. Bonnie, and R. L. Binder. "Resource Document on Mandatory Outpatient Treatment." *Journal of the American Academy of Psychiatry and the Law* 28, no. 2 (2000): 127–44.

Schwartz, Steven J., and Cathy E. Costanzo. "Compelling Treatment in the Community: Distorted Doctrines and Violated Values." *Loyola of Los Angeles Law Review* 20, no. 4 (June 1987): 1329–1429.

Swartz, M. S., and J. Monahan. "Special Section on Involuntary Outpatient Commitment: Introduction." *Psychiatric Services (Washington, D.C.)* 52, no. 3 (March 2001): 323–24.

Swartz, Marvin S., and Jeffrey W. Swanson. "Economic Grand Rounds: Can States Implement Involuntary Outpatient Commitment within Existing State Budgets?" *Psychiatric Services (Washington, D.C.)* 64, no. 1 (January 2013): 7–9. doi:10.1176/appi.ps.201200467.

Olmstead v. L.C. 527 US 581 (1999).

NRI Analytics. 2012. http://www.nri-incdata.org/ProfilesReport.cfm?Variable=T_4c3&State=All&Year=13&Description=How%20many%20total%20persons%20were%20under%20an%20outpatient%20commitment%20status%20in%20Fiscal%20Year%202012?&PTable=P13Involuntary.

Helping Families in Mental Health Crisis Act of 2013. HR 3717. https://www.congress.gov/bill/113th-congress/house-bill/3717/text.

Helping Families in Mental Health Crisis Act of 2015. HR 2646. https://www.congress.gov/bill/114th-congress/house-bill/2646/text.

Swanson, Jeffrey. "Outpatient Commitment as Crisis Driven Law." Lecture at Sheppard Pratt Health System, February 5, 2014.

17. Jack Lesser and Mental Health Courts

Baltimore City Mental Health Court. *Procedure Manual* (2005, rev. 2006–2007, 2014). Chapter 1.

Earley, Pete. *Crazy: A Father's Search through America's Mental Health Madness*. Penguin, 2007.

Mental Health Courts. 42 US Code 3796ii–7.

Anestis, Joye C., and Joyce L. Carbonell. "Stopping the Revolving Door: Effectiveness of Mental Health Court in Reducing Recidivism by Mentally Ill Offenders." *Psychiatric Services (Washington, D.C.)* 65, no. 9 (September 1, 2014): 1105-12. doi:10.1176/appi.ps.201300305.

Almquist, L., and E. Dodd. "Mental Health Courts: A Guide to Research-Informed Policy and Practice." New York: Council of State Governments Justice Center, 2009. https://www.bja.gov/Publications/CSG_MHC_Research.pdf.

McNiel, Dale E., Naomi Sadeh, Kevin L. Delucchi, and Renée L. Binder. "Prospective Study of Violence Risk Reduction by a Mental Health Court." *Psychiatric Services (Washington, D.C.)* 66, no. 6 (June 2015): 598–603. doi:10.1176/appi.ps.201400203.

Steadman, Henry J., Lisa Callahan, Pamela Clark Robbins, Roumen Vesselinov, Thomas G. McGuire, and Joseph P. Morrissey. "Criminal Justice and Behavioral Health Care Costs of Mental Health Court Participants: A Six-Year Study." *Psychiatric Services (Washington, D.C.)* 65, no. 9 (September 2014): 1100–104. doi:10.1176/appi.ps.201300375.

Stawicki, Elizabeth. "Study: Mental Health Court Showing Positive Results." *MPR News*, July 17, 2009. http://www.mprnews.org/story/2009/07/17/mental_health_courts.

Lamb, H. R. "Does Deinstitutionalization Cause Criminalization? The Penrose Hypothesis." *JAMA Psychiatry* 72, no. 2 (2015): 105–6. doi:10.1001/jamapsychiatry.2014.2444.

Steadman, Henry J., Allison Redlich, Lisa Callahan, Pamela Clark Robbins, and Roumen Vesselinov. "Effect of Mental Health Courts on Arrests and Jail Days: A Multisite Study." *Archives of General Psychiatry* 68, no. 2 (2011): 167–72. doi: 10.1001/archgenpsychiatry.2010.134.

18. Dan, Guns, and Mental Illness

Kessler, Ronald C., Patricia Berglund, Olga Demler, Robert Jin, Kathleen R. Merikangas, and Ellen E. Walters. "Lifetime Prevalence and Age-of-Onset Distributions of DSM-IV Disorders in the National Comorbidity Survey Replication." *Archives of General Psychiatry* 62, no. 6 (2005): 593–602.

Obama, Barack. Broadcast remarks, July 24, 2012. http://www.msnbc.com/the-ed-show/obama-ak-47s-belong-the-hands-so.

Holmes arsenal collection. January 2013. http://abcnews.go.com/blogs/headlines/2013/01/james-holmes-legally-bought-arsenal-of-guns-chemicals/.

Swanson, Jeffrey. Video of lecture, Stanford Law School, May 23, 2013. https://www.youtube.com/watch?v=5BGmcCo53Vo.

Gun Control Act of 1968. Public Law 90-618 (1968). https://www.gpo.gov/fdsys/pkg/STATUTE-82/pdf/STATUTE-82-Pg1213-2.pdf.

District of Columbia v. Heller. 128 S.Ct. 2783 (2008).

McDonald v. Chicago. 561 US 742 (2010).

Tyler v. Hillsdale County Sheriff's Department. US Court of Appeals for the Sixth Circuit. No. 13-1876 (2014). http://www.ca6.uscourts.gov/opinions.pdf/14a0296p-06.pdf.

New York SAFE Act (2013). http://www.omh.ny.gov/omhweb/safe_act/.

Health—General. Maryland Code Annotated §10-632. http://web.lexisnexis.com/research/xlink?app=00075&view=full&interface=1&docinfo=off&searchtype=get&search=Md.+HEALTH-GENERAL+Code+Ann.+%A7+10-632. Accessed January 24, 2016.

Warrant for Firearms or Ammunition in Control of Person Subject to Gun Violence Restraining Order. California Penal Code § 1542.5. http://www.leginfo.ca.gov/cgi-bin/displaycode?section=pen&group=01001-02000&file=1523-1542.5. Accessed January 24, 2016.

Welsh-Huggins, Andrew. "Attorney General Questions Court-Ordered Hospitalization Numbers." *Ohio.com*, August 25, 2013.

Dance, Scott, and Erin Cox. "Police: Perry Hall Shooting Suspect Knew of Step-Father's Gun Cache." *Baltimore Sun*, August 31, 2012.

Vittes, Katherine A., Daniel W. Webster, Shannon Frattaroli, Barbara E. Claire, and Garen J. Wintemute. "Removing Guns from Batterers: Findings from a Pilot Survey of Domestic Violence Restraining Order Recipients in California." *Violence against Women* 19, no. 5 (May 2013): 602–16. doi:10.1177/1077801213490561.

19. Bryan Stanley, Violence, and Psychiatric Illness

Torrey, E. Fuller. *The Insanity Offense: How America's Failure to Treat the Seriously Mentally Ill Endangers Its Citizens*. Norton, 2012.

Jungen, A. "Neighbors Say Bryan Stanley Was Quiet, Friendly." *La-Crosse Tribune*, March 15, 2012. http://lacrossetribune.com/news/local/neighbors-say-bryan-stanley-was-quiet-friendly/article_ffeb1b30-6e4f-11e1-9ded-001871e3ce6c.html.

Swanson, J. W., C. E. Holzer, V. K. Ganju, and R. T. Jono. "Violence and Psychiatric Disorder in the Community: Evidence from the Epidemiologic Catchment Area Surveys." *Hospital and Community Psychiatry* 41, no. 7 (July 1990): 761–70.

Van Dorn, Richard, Jan Volavka, and Norman Johnson. "Mental Disorder and Violence: Is There a Relationship beyond Substance Use?" *Social Psychiatry and Psychiatric Epidemiology* 47, no. 3 (March 2012): 487–503. doi:10.1007/s00127-011-0356-x.

Steadman, H. J., E. P. Mulvey, J. Monahan, P. C. Robbins, P. S. Appelbaum, T. Grisso, L. H. Roth, and E. Silver. "Violence by People Discharged from Acute Psychiatric Inpatient Facilities and by Others in the Same Neighborhoods." *Archives of General Psychiatry* 55, no. 5 (May 1998): 393–401.

Swanson, Jeffrey W., Marvin S. Swartz, Richard A. Van Dorn, Eric B. Elbogen, H. Ryan Wagner, Robert A. Rosenheck, T. Scott Stroup, Joseph P. McEvoy, and Jeffrey A. Lieberman. "A National Study of Violent Behavior in Persons with Schizophrenia." *Archives of General Psychiatry* 63, no. 5 (May 2006): 490–99. doi:10.1001/archpsyc.63.5.490.

Torrey, E. Fuller, Jonathan Stanley, John Monahan, and Henry J. Steadman, MacArthur Study Group. "The MacArthur Violence Risk Assessment Study Revisited: Two Views Ten Years after Its Initial Publication." *Psychiatric Services (Washington, D.C.)* 59, no. 2 (February 2008): 147–52. doi:10.1176/appi.ps.59.2.147.

Skeem, J., P. Kennealy, J. Monahan, J. Peterson, and P. Appelbaum. "Psychosis Uncommonly and Inconsistently Precedes Violence among High-Risk Individuals." *Clinical Psychological Science* (April 24, 2015). doi:10.1177/2167702615575879.

Lidz, C. W., E. P. Mulvey, and W. Gardner. "The Accuracy of Predictions of Violence to Others." *Journal of the American Medical Association* 269, no. 8 (February 1993): 1007–11.

Monahan, John. "Dangerousness and Disorder: Requiring Treatment to Attenuate Risk." Lecture presented at a Scattergood Foundation applied ethics workshop "Dangerousness and Involuntary Treatment," University of Pennsylvania, March 19, 2014.

State v. Stanley. 762 N.W.2d 864 (2008).

State v. Stanley. Wisconsin Court of Appeals, unpublished opinion. Appeal no. 2012AP1558-CR (2013).

Stanley v. Van Rybroek. US District Court for the Western District of Wisconsin. Opinion and Order 14-cv-181-wmc (2015).

20. Amy and Involuntary Treatment for Suicide Prevention

Mental Health Reporting. "Facts about Mental Illness and Suicide." http://depts .washington.edu/mhreport/facts_suicide.php.

Dahlberg, Linda L., Robin M. Ikeda, and Marcie-Jo Kresnow. "Guns in the Home and Risk of a Violent Death in the Home: Findings from a National Study." *American Journal of Epidemiology* 160, no. 10 (November 2004): 929–36. doi:10.1093/aje/kwh309.

Rosen, David H. "Suicide Survivors: A Follow-Up Study of Persons Who Survived Jumping from the Golden Gate and San Francisco Oakland Bay Bridges." *Western Journal of Medicine* 122, no. 4 (1975): 289–94.

Ruiz v. Estelle. 503 F.Supp. 1265 (1980).

Hanson, Annette. "Correctional Suicide: Has Progress Ended?" *Journal of the American Academy of Psychiatry and the Law* 38, no. 1 (2010): 6–10.

21. Will Forcing Treatment on People with Psychiatric Disorders Prevent Mass Murders?

Murphy, T. "Sandy Hook, Two Years Later: Politicians Owe It to the Families to Do Something." *Guardian*, December 14, 2014. http://www.theguardian.com /commentisfree/2014/dec/14/sandy-hook-two-years-later-politicians-mental -health.

Bjelopera, J., et al. *Public Mass Shootings in the United States: Selected Implications for Federal Public Health and Safety Policy.* Washington, DC: Congressional Research Service, 2013. https://www.fas.org/sgp/crs/misc/R43004.pdf.

Follman, Mark, Gavin Aronsen, and Deanna Pan. "US Mass Shootings, 1982–2016: Data from Mother Jones' Investigation." *Mother Jones.* http://www.motherjones .com/politics/2012/12/mass-shootings-mother-jones-full-data.

Blair, J. Pete, and Katherine W. Schweit. *A Study of Active Shooter Incidents, 2000–2013.* Washington, DC: Texas State University and Federal Bureau of Investigation, US Department of Justice, 2014.

Hempel, A. G., J. R. Meloy, and T. C. Richards. "Offender and Offense Characteristics of a Nonrandom Sample of Mass Murderers." *Journal of the American Academy of Psychiatry and the Law* 27, no. 2 (1999): 213–25.

Meloy, J. Reid, Anthony G. Hempel, B. Thomas Gray, Kris Mohandie, Andrew Shiva, and Thomas C. Richards. "A Comparative Analysis of North American Adolescent and Adult Mass Murderers." *Behavioral Sciences and the Law* 22, no. 3 (2004): 291–309. doi:10.1002/bsl.586.

Office of the Child Advocate. "Shooting at Sandy Hook Elementary School." November 22, 2014. http://www.nytimes.com/interactive/2014/11/22/nyregion /report-on-adam-lanza.html?_r=0.

Frosh, D. "James Holmes's Psychiatrist Testifies in Colorado Theater Shooting Trial." *Wall Street Journal*, June 16, 2015. http://www.wsj.com/articles/james-holmes -psychiatrist-testifies-in-colorado-theater-shooting-trial-1434484324.

"Mass Shootings at Virginia Tech: Report of the Review Panel." April 16, 2007. https://governor.virginia.gov/media/3772/fullreport.pdf.

Helping Families in Mental Health Crisis Act of 2013. HR 3717. https://www .congress.gov/bill/113th-congress/house-bill/3717/text.

Strengthening Mental Health in Our Communities Act of 2014. HR 4574. https:// www.congress.gov/bill/113th-congress/house-bill/4574.

Helping Families in Mental Health Crisis Act of 2015. HR 2646. https://www .congress.gov/bill/114th-congress/house-bill/2646/text.

22. Transforming the Battleground

"Getting Started." National Resource Center on Psychiatric Advance Directives. http://www.nrc-pad.org/getting-started. Accessed July 12, 2015.

"Psychiatric Advance Directives." Bazelon Center for Mental Health Law. http:// www.bazelon.org/Where-We-Stand/Self-Determination/Advance-Directives .aspx. Accessed July 12, 2015.

"Medicare Resident Limits." Association of American Medical Colleges. https:// www.aamc.org/advocacy/gme/71178/gme_gme0012.html. Accessed July 12, 2015.

"Physician Supply and Demand: Projections to 2020." US Department of Health and Human Services. October 2006. http://bhpr.hrsa.gov/healthworkforce /supplydemand/medicine/physician2020projections.pdf.

Insel, Thomas. "Anatomy of NIMH Funding." http://www.nimh.nih.gov/funding/ funding-strategy-for-research-grants/white-paper_149362.pdf. Accessed July 12, 2015.

"ACA and State Governments: Consider Savings as Well as Costs." Robert Wood Johnson Foundation Urban Institute. http://www.urban.org/research/public ation/aca-and-state-governments-consider-savings-well-costs. Accessed July 15, 2015.

Buck, David S., Carlie A. Brown, and J. Scott Hickey. "The Jail Inreach Project: Linking Homeless Inmates Who Have Mental Illness with Community Health Services." *Psychiatric Services (Washington, D.C.)* 62, no. 2 (February 2011): 120–22. doi:10.1176/appi.ps.62.2.120.

Brown, Carlie A., J. Scott Hickey, and David S. Buck. "Shaping the Jail Inreach Project: Program Evaluation as a Quality Improvement Measure to Inform Programmatic Decision Making and Improve Outcomes." *Journal of Health Care for the Poor and Underserved* 24, no. 2 (2013): 435–43. doi:10.1353/hpu.2013.0063.

Index